Providing Health Care For Individuals With Intellectual Disability And Mental Health Conditions In Rural Settings: *Problems, Practice, And Progress*

Edited by John Holderegger, M.S. & Ann R. Poindexter, M.D.

NADD An association for persons with developmental disabilities and mental health needs.

132 Fair Street
Kingston, NY 12401

LCCN: 2006936143
ISBN: 1-57256-045-2

Printed in the United States of America

Table of Contents

Foreword v

Culture of Rural America: Impact on Health Services 1

History and Outcome of Various Approaches:
Mental Health Services in a Rural Prairie State 17

Coming Home on the Range:
Changing Profiles of the People Served and the
Provision of Their Community and Institutional Services
in Rural Wyoming, 1988-2004 33

Community Support Teams:
A Collaborative Home-Based Support Model 51

Living Well with CMS Funding: A Study of Mortality in Wyoming 65

Fiscal Issues:
Predicting Individual Budgets in a Support Program
for People with Developmental Disabilities: An Evaluation. 75

Building Wyoming Developmental Disability Waivers:
Stewardship for the 21st Century 95

Specific Programs and Approaches:
Working Together for Success:
Enlisting and Training Staff in Dual Diagnosis 101

Wyoming Works to Preserve Major Improvements in
Retention by Enhancing Wages and Training 105

Specific Programs and Approaches:
Telehealth in Rural America 109

Rural Psychotherapy and Developmental Disability. 117

Domestic Violence:
Supporting Women to Live Safely in Community Settings in Alaska. 131

Foreword

Those who work with those persons with developmental disabilities who have a co-occurring mental illness and live in a rural area are acutely aware of the inherent difficulty of getting all the services these persons need, especially finding the service provider(s) with the expertise necessary to deal with their specialized needs as dictated by their co-occurring disabilities. Many communities in rural areas are fairly skilled at dealing with someone who has by definition a singular issue of a developmental disability. Most have gotten these skills due to this individual being born and raised in the area or being returned to the area after the downsizing of a state institution. Nevertheless, even the smallest community or rural area has been able to compensate fairly well for this individual. And many can handle the challenges brought forward by the individual who has a bona fide mental illness. But when someone with a dual diagnosis arrives on the scene, the single purpose provider is not equipped to handle the challenge.

Enough cannot be said about the detail and thoroughness of the individual plan of care. Individuals who have co-occurring disabilities need to have a structured plan of care that leaves little or no flexibility to the person's life. For the individual to feel in control the plan must be applied consistently and, where possible, be implemented by the same people. Havoc and change are the two worst enemies to these persons with a dual diagnosis being able to live and thrive in rural environments. It is essential that a detailed behavioral intervention plan be individualized and consistently implemented in order to give the person served a sense of control and consistency. We find that acting out behaviorally can be tied directly back to a lack of consistent plan implementation. The individual with dual diagnosis feels that he or she is losing control and acts out to bring more control back into his or her life.

When serving persons with the co-occurring disabilities of developmental disabilities and mental illness it is important to think "outside the box" and use non-traditional solutions to solve problems. With *Olmstead vs. L.C.* looming over the states' heads and with deinstitutionalization resulting in more persons with more severe disabilities entering rural environments as well as more urban areas, it is essential that the interdisciplinary teams not only understand the limitations of such placement, but also the rich opportunities that exist there as well.

This book is dedicated to all those persons with co-occurring developmental disabilities and mental illness who choose to live in the rural areas of the world and to those who dedicate their lives to making these citizens' lives worth living. As we put these chapters together we have become more and more excited about some of the very innovative projects that are going on in some <u>very</u> remote areas—we feel that even those who work in <u>very</u> urban areas can learn from this material. The problems we all face are exceptionally complex, and we can, indeed, learn a lot from each other!

We particularly want to thank those from North Carolina, Alaska, North Dakota,

Louisiana, California, Oregon, Arkansas, Colorado, and Wyoming who have authored chapters for this book, as well as the informal input we've received from many other rural areas around North America. The various chapters we've included address both adminstrative and clinical issues.

John Holderegger, M.S. & Ann R. Poindexter, M.D.

Culture of Rural America: Impact on Health Services

Jarrett Barnhill, M.D., University of North Carolina School of Medicine

Introduction

There are many issues that affect the availability and utilization of services for individuals with intellectual disability and mental disorders. In rural settings, demographic, geographic, and local economic factors are frequently cited as barriers to community-based programs (Bouras, Brooks, & Drummond, 1994; Braddock, Hemp, & Rizzolo, 2004). The changing age-demographics of many rural communities helps illustrate this point. These age-related changes grew out of improvements in health care, and the end result was a steady growth in the numbers of older citizens in many rural areas (Smith, 1997). A significant increase in the longevity of people with developmental disabilities has also occurred. As a result of these demographic changes there are increasing pressures on service delivery systems to accommodate both of these age-related issues (Smith, 1997; Haley, 2004; Janicki, McCallion, Force, Bishop, & LeProe, 1998)

For individuals with intellectual disabilities, these age-related demographic changes create a paradox. Aging parents mean an inevitable decline in the most prevalent form of placement, home-based care (Haley, 2004; Young & Ashamn, 2004). At the same time, increased longevity of individuals with intellectual disability (ID) means that services are needed for a longer period of time. The paradox emerges when the advantages provided by improved medical care end up creating a new problem—increasing numbers of people with ID who are losing their primary placement. In other words the demand for caregivers was growing as the supply of traditional system of caregivers (extended families) was shrinking. In addition, the increasing needs for specialized health care needed by an older population are further straining both community-based and residential programs as well. The out-migration of young people compounds the problem by decreasing the pool of younger relatives who will take over the care of intellectually disabled siblings and close relatives (Haley, 2004; Heller & Factor, 1993; Llewellyn, Gething, Kendig, & Cant, 2004).

Both an aging population and loss of traditional caregivers was especially problematic for many of those with psychiatric disorders, which put many families in the unenviable position of choosing between long term placement, dealing with repeated psychiatric hospitalizations, or struggling to make at home a form of de facto institution—the family becomes institutionalized in its own home by the individual's illness (Haley & Perkins, 2004; Greenblatt, 1976; Reeve, Aceves, Morrales, Thorne-Lehman, & Vickers, 1998; Young & Ashamn, 2004)

This chapter will explore the cultural and psychosocial forces that influence the availability and use of community services, but in order to understand the effects of culture, we first need to consider both the structure (ideals and value system) and function of institutions (role of schools, churches, etc.) germane to a community's way of doing things. We will explore the effects of ever-changing realities such as the effects of social change on local services needs, availability of community-based programs, and utilization of these resources. As we shall see, defining rural in terms of culture and culture change paints a far more complex picture than one that relies solely on economic or geographic factors (Prunchno, Patrick, & Burant, 2004).

What Is The Problem?

The most commonly cited reasons for placement outside of the community include disruptive or aggressive behaviors, availability of an appropriate level of care, and effectiveness of existing services (Brunnicks, Thurlow, Thurman, & Forelli, 1980; Magana, Seltzer, & Kraus, 2002). The placement decision reflects a balance between these factors and the carrying capacity of existing community institutions (Dean, 1976; Barnhill & Barnhill, 2002; Lewis-Fernandez & Kleinman, 1995). Carrying capacity represents a balance between factors such as the number of affected people, severity of their problems, and the capacity of the community to tolerate or willingness to deal with these problems. In rural areas, carrying capacity can be compromised by inadequate transportation to distant treatment programs (service availability). A lack of transportation means that fewer people can access services. As a result, families are left outside the service loop, and respite, workshop, or day treatment may not be available. Lacking these services many families may feel over-burdened and less tolerant of their developmentally disabled relative. These problems may translate into a lowered threshold for placement outside the community (Dean, 1976; Smith, 1997; Young & Ashamn, 2004)

In addition to issues of availability, low utilization rates of available services also affect carrying capacity. Utilization rates tend to reflect attitudes (value system) towards or willingness (e.g. belief in efficacy or stigmatization) to use local community-based programs (Pruncho & McMullen 2004). For caregivers, utilization relates to education level, poverty, political and social conservatism, attitudes towards mental illness, and discomfort with "government" imposed programs (Barnhill & Barnhill, 2002).

It is apparent from this list that cultural factors also play a significant role in service use and carrying capacity (Brunnicks et al., 1980). For many communities, traditional patterns of dealing with individuals with ID differed from those needed for individuals with severe mental disorders. Under these circumstances local attitudes and theories about the causes of severe behavioral problems/psychiatric disorders had a major impact on carrying capacity. In other words, tolerance for severe aggression in the context of schizophrenia may be far lower than it is for stereotypic behaviors in a person with "uncomplicated" ID. Unfortunately for people with dual diagnoses, low carrying capacity meant an even lower threshold for placement, traditionally in a state-run hospital or ICF/MR facility (Knobbe, Carey, Rhodes, & Horner, 1995; Young & Ashamn, 2004).

Who Lives in Rural America?

There are many rural Americas. Even though many rural people share similar social, political, and religious values, there are considerable differences in how culture, geography, and underlying economic forces shape their world-view (Braddock, Hemp, & Rizzolo, 2004; Lakin, Pouty, & Coucouvanis, 2004). The recent presidential election reflects some of this diversity. Even though the majority of "red states" are demographically rural and politically conservative, there is considerable intra-state variability in attitudes and values that affect local, state, congressional, and senatorial elections. Likewise, many states in the "blue" column also have large rural populations for which agriculture and ranching account for a substantial portion of local economies. The rural or "bubba factor" plays a significant role in local affairs that are frequently in step with the view that "all politics is local."

These diverse findings suggest that no single set of values and attitudes reflects rural America in its entirety. So which features best describe "rural America"? Researchers frequently rely on population density to define "rural." Based on this definition, rural areas should have fewer people spread out over larger geographic areas. Put another way, there are greater distances between people and fewer high-density places like cities. As a result, services are also scattered over a larger geographic area, and access to medical and/or mental health care may require traveling substantial distances. Low population densities may also decrease the likelihood that specialized services will be accessible or available in many rural settings (Turner, 1998; Fox, Blank, Rovnyak, & Barnett, 2001; Heller, 1993; Gurwitt, 1998).

There is a longstanding history of out-migration of young people from most rural communities resulted in significant changes in age-demographics. The emigration of rural children contributed not only to a brain drain but also disrupted many informal and traditional networks of caregivers or support systems. The rising mean age in many rural areas also reflects this migration. Even though population density was not changed significantly, the aging rural population created a growing concentration of land rich-cash poor individuals who tended to be high users of community services. In spite of their greater need for services, the remaining older folks were also more likely to share negative attitudes about taxes to fund programs and to be wary of many federal programs (Turner, 1998; Fox et al., 2001; Heller & Factor, 1993).

These demographic changes indirectly affect the availability of services– the "safety net" is stretched thin. The increased ratio of the elderly to younger workers also results in fewer local financial resources. These socio-economic trends make it difficult to provide extensive (and expensive) state-of-the-art services especially for people who are dually diagnosed.

At a practical level, the loss of extended families can directly limit access to services—the cousin or neighbor is no longer able to provide transportation. This shift resulted in an increased reliance on church "family", "the government", or more formalized/contractual services. Unfortunately, the dependence on more formalized providers increased the potential for conflicts between attitudes of self-sufficiency, not trusting "government programs," "not wanting to be a burden," or discomfort with (or suspiciousness of) bureaucratized, government services (Smith, 1997; Johnson, Beale, Gurwitt, & Turner, 2000; Reed, 1974).

Out of necessity, many rural families eventually end up relying on governmental services in spite of feeling handicapped by limited education or a lack of bureaucratic "street smarts." As a result, there is ample opportunity for conflicts between what the families feel is fair or needed and the impersonal rules, regulations, and legal restraints required by these programs. The stage is set for conflicts between locals that may adversely affect service utilization (Warner, 1985; Llewellyn, Gething, Kendig, & Cant, 2004; Prunchno et al., 1997; Patterson & Friel, 2001).

In summary, the extent to which these issues impede service utilization has more to do with social and cultural factors than geographic distance or population density. Regardless of source, there are many roadblocks to providing services for people with intellectual disability (ID) in general and dual diagnosis in particular. In fact services for individuals with dual diagnoses may be most sensitive to socio-cultural and economic forces (Braddock et al., 2004; Rizzolo, Hemp, Braddock, & Pomeranz-Essley, 2004).

Economics and Psychological Geography

The majority of rural people either live in the countryside or in small towns. Socioeconomically, many of these communities represent extensions of the surrounding countryside—farm dwellers also working in town and town folks working on farms or ranches. Historically, living in a rural area also generally defined one's livelihood. Traditional sources of livelihood include farming, ranching, fishing, or other extractive industries, and their supporting industries (e.g. agribusiness) (Reed, 1993a; 1993b).

In the past, many small towns also had local department stores, a town physician, many churches, and, in the rural south, a caste system that segregated whites from African-Americans. Individuals were often defined in relation to their extended family, what church they belonged to, where they were raised, or for "outsiders," how long they have lived in the area. In most small communities, social and economic transactions were cemented by these extensive kinship or local community networks. As a result of these extensive ties, local economies operated on a more informal-personal basis, with less emphasis placed on legal contracts or formalized roles (Reed, 1974).

In many rural communities, the informal network of institutional supports also included schools and local churches. These organizations provided not only for educational and religious needs, they also provide a second layer of informal community supports. In many small towns, ministers joined the ranks of teachers and physicians as the "educated" folks. Traditionally the "smart folks" played a role in many local decisions and provided advice to others (paternalism). For example, local physicians were considered in more informal psychological terms. This sense of respectful obedience or deference differed from the more formalized, contractual, and even collaborative "modern" doctor-patient relationship. As a result of paternalistic attitudes, the opinions of these local educated folks had a greater influence on decisions about a child with intellectual disability. If these leaders supported placement, then the family might feel more pressure to acquiesce to place their child or family member outside the community. It was tacitly assumed that these folks knew what was best, and many people trusted that the professionals knew what they were talking about (Barnhill & Barnhill, 2002; Reed, 1993a; 1993b).

The complex relationship between place and psyche helped solidify a sense of psychological geography. As a result of geographic attachment, many local folks had a feeling that their local store or school, no matter how far behind the objective standards of outsiders, was superior to the one in the next town or county (Reed, 1974). In this context, stores, schools, and residential institutions are closely linked to attitudes about the meaning of location and prevailing ways of doing things. From this perspective the sense of possessing land or structures assumed a much deeper significance than dirt or bricks. Many small communities evolved into small psychological city-states where the sense of psychological place gave special status to the "home place," farm, or "home town." This feeling seemed to be especially strong in areas where many people spent most of their lives in the same house or area where generations of relatives were born and lived out their lives (Barnhill & Barnhill, 2002; Reed, 1993b).

For rural southerners, the lifestyle of even the most impoverished regions was superior to that of any urban environment, particularly anything from "up north." This attitude (regionalism) applied to differences within a state (mountains versus piedmont or coast), city-country ("city folks don't understand our ways"), or larger geographic areas. The regional biases produce interesting results. For example, people from rural California, New York, New Mexico, or Alaska are considered in the same light as local folks. People from areas surrounding large metropolitan areas are considered to be different, especially if they are educated, affluent, and "not like us." This sense of regional ethnocentrism continues even though these contested regions are clearly rural and have a similar economy based on agriculture or ranching. In many circumstances these attitudes persist in spite of objective measures that do not support marked differences in social institutions or other attitudinal systems (Johnson et al., 2000; Reed, 1974; 1993a; 1993b).

Unfortunately this sort of local ethnocentrism (regionalism) can create real barriers to change. For example, local folks might not appreciate opinions or solutions to "our" problems—especially those coming from outsiders who are just "pretending" to be country folks. Regardless of merit, suggestions from "experts" (including advocates and reformers) might be considered as unsuitable for "our people."

"Where Have All the Young Men (and Women) Gone?"

Out-migration of young people is one of the root causes of the population loss in many rural communities. Most moved to metropolitan and then suburban places looking for jobs, education, culture, and better lives for themselves and their families. Unfortunately many of these young people represented the better-educated, highly skilled, or ambitious young people. This change in population dynamics created problems due not only to lost income and local tax revenues, but also left behind an aging remnant with greater health needs (Johnson et al., 2000).

For African Americans, there were multiple waves of migrations beginning in the latter part of the 19th century and extending through both World Wars. There were many underlying motives for this migration. Most immigrants left for a better life and economic opportunities in the urban "north" and to escape racism, "Jim Crow" laws, and *de jure* segregation in the south. The great migrations resulted in a significant demographic shift as African Americans became an increasingly urbanized ethnic group. The remnant of African-Americans remaining in the predominantly agrarian south remained under Jim Crow laws and a caste system (Meier, 1969; Ossofsky, 1969; Klarman, 2003).

In spite of some movement into the middle class, poverty, crime, "ghetto-ization," and other urban ills complicated the acculturation of many African-Americans. As an outlet, many urbanites maintained contacts with their rural extended families. It was a common practice for their many families to send children for the summers to stay with grandparents—troubled youth were also sent to relatives to get them "off the streets." These "urbanized" children returned with very different attitudes about the racial caste system and other aspects of segregation—often with tragic consequences. Even though this contact was not a major contributor, the movement of African-Americans played a role in both the growth of the civil rights movement and the violent backlash unleashed by southern racists—who always cited the negative effects of outside, "northern" agitators on our "happy colored people" (Prunchno 1997; Klarman, 2003).

"You Can Go Home Again?"

The trend towards out-migration may be changing, as new immigrants are moving into rural communities. One motivation is disillusionment with urban and suburban life—an outgrowth of the "back-to-nature" movement and an attempt to escape "toxic effects" of urban environments (Duany, Plater-Zybek, & Speck, 2000; Turner, 1998). Recent technological advances such as better transportation and telecommuting are playing key roles. Many "techies" can now work in rural settings. Although the numbers are smaller than previous out-migrations, the movement (or return of children) of technologically sophisticated young people is having an impact on existing age-income demographics. In some respects, this influx of these relatively affluent young people resembles urban "gentrification." "Gentrification" is also associated with increased day-to-day contact between middle class, highly educated, professionals and local folks. These new people ("yankees" to many die-hard southerners) are bringing a different life-style and demanding a wider variety of educational experiences and consumer-entertainment preferences. In essence, they are bringing "urban" cultural values with them (Turner, 1998; Johnson et al., 2000; Reed, 1993a).

Latino immigrations present a more fluid process. People in many rural counties are accustomed to the essential role latinos play in seasonal agriculture. As a result many rural counties have long experiences with transient changes in their hispanic populations. In recent years, there is a growing permanent Latino presence that is expressed in rapidly growing nonagricultural job opportunities. Acculturation is affected by language differences, forcing many rural areas to accommodate or adapt to a Spanish-speaking or bilingual community. For example, schools, social agencies, and health care providers are providing Spanish-language materials. The permanent Latino community is shifting the demographics of many rural counties. Cultural influences are also growing. Spanish language radio stations, churches, and other cultural events are becoming more prominent. Latinos are also bringing different traditions about the roles of family, professionals and other government programs in the care of individuals with intellectual disabilities and mental disorders (Lewis-Fernandez & Kleinman, 1995; Burnette, 2000).

In addition to immigrants from urban centers, many younger African-Americans are also choosing to remain in rural areas (Meier, 1969; Prunchno, Patrick, & Brant, 1997). Some of this change may reflect increasing opportunities or frustrations with urban lifestyles. The growing strength of an urban black middle class is impacting not only southern cities such as Atlanta, but also many smaller communities in the hinterlands. For city-dwellers, dissatisfaction with urban environments is increasing the likelihood of a different pattern of rural migration (intra-regional). The impact of this migration is still being felt as new arrivals make adjustments to the differences between an urban culture and more conservative rural areas (Klarman, 2003). The interaction between these arrivals and locals will be a complex process. The interface and potential value conflicts between these new immigrants and local folks will play out in the struggles for adequate services for individuals with dual diagnoses (Klarman, 2003).

The old pattern of poor aging rural folks is changing as the result of a reverse migration associated with the booming market for retirement communities. This is changing economic-cultural demographics in selected areas. Many of these retirees are better educated and often substantially wealthier than the natives. They also bring a different set of attitudes regarding taxation, politics, medical care, and social programs. There is little data on the impact of these "gray" migrants (no longer just snow birds) on community attitudes towards other public programs for people with dual diagnoses—e.g. willingness to pay local property or other taxes to support school systems or programs for those with developmental disabilities. Those older Americans who have children with disabilities may have a different perspective, and will struggle to find services. Although there is limited supporting data, this group may be far more "militant" in pushing communities to develop appropriate services (Heller & Factor, 1993; Johnson et al., 2000).

A poignant variation on this theme involves the return of many former émigrés with HIV or end-stage AIDS—from either IV drug abuse or from homosexual or "promiscuous" heterosexual relationships (Berry, 1993; Cohn, Mohr, & Weber, 1994). It is ironic that some gays who originally escaped rural communities for sexual freedom returned home for care. For these individuals, returning home with AIDS meant "coming out the closet" at multiple levels. Many returned at a time when homosexuality and AIDS were stigmatized and some religious communities considered their illness to be punishment for their sins. Most rural communities were unprepared for both medical care and psychological needs of this disease (Berry, 1993; National Rural Health Association, 2004).

The response of rural communities to HIV/AIDS provides an example of problems rural folks experience in resource allocation. Beginning in the mid 1990's the number of HIV/AIDs cases increased significantly in rural/non-urban counties. Although social and cultural factors contributed to this rise in reported cases, access to medical professionals willing to work with AIDS patients, location of clinics specializing in the complex treatment regimens, and limited social support systems created problems. In many regions public health departments became the central point for evaluation and treatment, but many individuals remained reluctant to use these facilities because of concerns with privacy, low levels of awareness, and socio-religious conflicts (National Rural Health Association, 2004).

Each of these examples also points to the diverse challenges facing rural communities. It is apparent that the effects of demographic change (population density, age of returnees, etc.) are complex and that the changing definition of "rural" is not amenable to simple models. It is also apparent thus far that neither population density nor distance from metropolitan areas predicts a specific value system or pattern of thinking.

We need to explore the effects of these new arrivals on traditional ways of relating and care giving. Although an entirely different problem, developing services for AIDS patients may have many parallels to creating programs for individuals with dual diagnoses. For both, there is a shortage of services and a shrinking pool of traditional caregivers. This parallel may be more obvious for people with ID and mental disorders returning from institutional care settings.

There are potential conflicts with locals based on the many attitudinal differences these new urbanized "immigrants" bring with them. These newcomers and even adult children returning "home" may not understand or be willing to provide in-home care like their parents or grandparents did. They may also be unwilling to rebuild the informal network of family based-care. But these "newbies" may be more willing to invest in community-based professional services and support replacing these traditional ways of handling those with ID/MI with more innovative but more formal programs (Barnhill & Barnhill, 2002; Fox, Merwin, & Blank, 1995; Fox et al., 2001; Haley & Perkins, 2004).

"The Times They Are A Changin'"

Realistically, few rural communities ever come close to media portrayals of happy communities, filled with folks who are wise and noble, "picking and grinning," folksy, contented, genteel, and friendly. A reality check reveals that many rural areas are plagued by poverty, mental disorders, violence, and substance abuse. The not-so-bucolic reality is a reflection of many factors, but recent social changes are playing an ongoing role (Fox et al., 1995; Fox et al., 2001; Turner, 1998). This reality also challenges regional ethnocentric views about the superiority of local, small town, or rural institutions (regionalism). Local reactions to these challenges were played out in many arenas (education, local economies, and health care) and force us to address the impact of culture change.

In many rural communities there is a considerable education gap in standardized measures of academic performance between their rural school district and those from more affluent cities and suburbs. In order to close the gap and better prepare children to compete in a 21st century economy, school boards and local citizens voted to consolidate into bigger facilities. Unfortunately educational reform like other moves towards centralization and economies of scale carried a price. One of the negative consequences (unanticipated in many communities) of the closing of small community schools was a fundamental shift in the functional role of schools in the local culture. Consolidated, county schools made it more difficult to maintain older, informal, social institutions (Reed, 1974; 1993a; 1993b). They were too big and bureaucratized to maintain the personal touches that cemented an earlier sense of psychological geography.

The out-migration of upwardly mobile and frequently more highly educated young people resulted in shortages of farm workers—aside from Latino migrants. These changes along with increased operating costs, mechanization, and demands for greater productivity contributed to a consolidation of farm operations and disappearance of many family farms. For many rural communities, the emergence of corporate farms and ranches dismantled a way of life and the close network of social/economic interrelationships that was the lifeblood of many rural communities. The loss of "land" also further undermined the psychological sense of place (psychological geography) (Gurwitt, 1998; Kessler, 2000).

A similar challenge awaited other local commerce—local stores. The invasion of national or international retailers into small communities also changed the face of local economies. For most rural communities, the price for greater access to a wider variety of goods and services meant a trend towards greater regionalization of shopping. Chains of superstores replaced local, family-owned businesses. These changes have a significant impact on local economies, shifting the distribution of services and retail merchants from small town to regional centers. As a result many small towns face not only declining population but also shifts in tax base. The old ways of informal business and social relationships are also dying out (Turner, 1998; Gurwitt, 1998).

The relative depopulation and shift in traditional social and economic relationships also meant changes in social and health care services. For many smaller communities, medical care would become increasingly regionalized, as large group practices, HMOs, and an increasing array of "specialists" replaced the town "doc." Communities that still had health care professionals struggled to keep their physicians. Many community hospitals closed. These changes occurred in spite of substantial efforts to train physicians in family medicine or other primary care specialties. Although helpful in increasing the number of physician/unit population, many programs are still geographically concentrated into regional or hospital-medical center complexes. This centralization of treatment resources added geographic distance to already existing cultural or ethnic concerns over "modern" medicine (Warner, 1985; Anderson, 1995).

These cultural forces have an even greater impact on mental health services. Even though traditional healers or clergy may ease the burden, there are still substantial gaps between the quality and availability of psychiatrists, psychologists, or other mental health professionals. Ongoing efforts to restructure rural mental health services in many states have run into the problems with maldistribution of mental health professionals. The impact of many mental health reform movements may further limit the availability of local services. Many states are turning to private service provider networks but many are unwilling or unable to close the gaps (Kleinman, 1988; Fox et al., 1995; Fox et al., 2001).

Another factor is the culture of mental health services. Many mental health professionals are trained at major universities and have limited clinical experience with rural people, tenant farmers, or ranch hands. For many professionals there is a cultural dissonance between their scientific or theoretical training and local beliefs and theories about mental disorders. One solution to closing the cultural gap is using indigenous mental health workers or recruiting professionals who will live in rural settings (Fox et al., 1995; Fox et al., 2001; Johnson et al., 2000; Kessler, 2000).

But this option is more complicated than it seems. Many mental health clinicians prefer a sense of community with other professionals, and tend to create small islands or communities within a community. These factors may partly explain the tendency for clinicians to cluster in population centers where they can find or more readily develop a supportive professional community.

Technology may provide a solution. Teleconferencing can be used to compensate for professional isolation, provide ongoing consultation, and shorten the time required for assessments (decrease transit time). But there are limits to technology. Many mental health functions require close contact. At present there is limited evidence that these advances will dramatically accelerate the influx of or acculturation of young professionals to rural settings (Kleinman, 1988; Fox et al.,

1995; Greenblatt, 1976; Kessler, 2000). The underlying issues affecting acculturation and belonging to a place still remain—I don't think I have ever heard some one referred as the "town" psychiatrist or psychologist.

These problems are compounded at all levels for clinicians who work in the field of dual diagnosis. In most settings there is a regional mix of local services and profit, nonprofit, and state supported programs. By necessity and low population density, many of these programs are regionalized and access to mental health or medical care is frequently geographically dispersed. Because expertise is so limited, we need to expand the use of these new technologies to deal with issues of professional as well as geographic isolation (Bouras et al., 1994; Menolascino, 1994; Magana et al., 2002; Young & Ashamn, 2004).

Culture Change and Rural Service Delivery

In order to understand the dynamic of culture change it may be helpful to look carefully at the process of adapting to culture change. First of all, culture change is multi-dimensional and nonlinear. In theory, the dominant culture (technologically advanced or better armed) has the greatest influence. Within the U.S. there are many competing forces and multi-directional influences on social change. The most intriguing expression of multi-directional change involves the mass media exposure, TV, radio, music, etc. As a result of information sharing and the universal appeal of TV, we are witnessing the rise in popularity of NASCAR in traditionally urban settings and "hip-hop," rap, and salsa among rural southern whites (Barnhill & Barnhill, 2002; Reed, 1974; 1993a; 1993b).

Another approach to understanding culture change relies on an historical perspective. For example, the introduction of electricity, radio, television, and even the opening of the community's first fast food restaurant brought significant social changes to rural life. Manifestations of even newer technologies are everywhere–personal computers, Palm Pilots, high tech farm machinery, and a range of scientific instruments used by many younger farmers and ranchers. Although many locals may embrace technological change, they remain politically and culturally conservative (Turner, 1998; Gurwitt, 1998).

From a slightly different perspective, social change is unsettling for rural folks and can be met with a mixture of open acceptance and subtle resistance. On the negative side, social change is also associated with increases in stress-related diseases, substance abuse, violent behavior, and psychiatric disorders associated with social change. For others, there is an increase in conservative political or religious views. Conservative social and political views play out in attitudes about government-sponsored services, efforts to limit taxes of any sort and fatalistic attitudes towards mental illness and developmental disabilities, affecting access to or the availability of community-based services. Religious conservatism often emerges in waves such as the "great awakenings" (described later). It becomes readily apparent that in many rural settings, these belief sets (attitudinal differences) may be more important than low population density or geographic isolation (Kleinman, 1988; Lewis-Fernandez & Kleinman, 1995; Cash, 1941).

The widespread migrations from rural areas reflect earlier social, economic and technological changes. The inevitable effect of this migration was a loss of young people and a depopulation of extended families. The migrations then helped create a gap in the traditional, informal safety net support system in many rural settings. These traditional family-based support systems had played a key role in assisting families to coping with the "burdens" of a mentally ill intellectually disabled member. Their loss resulted in a serious erosion of the carrying capacity of these communities. The end result was a lower threshold or tolerance for aberrant behavior and a growing willingness for caregivers to rely on more restrictive solutions. These restrictive solutions were state run "institutions" (Warner, 1985; Knobbe et al.,1995; Noll, 1995). Unfortunately, once an individual was placed, many families then struggled with custodial programs that lacked habilitation services or that used excessive medication. The other option was not much better, staying at home and dealing with inadequately funded community mental health programs. Because many local programs also lacked appropriate programs, families could be ensnared by another vicious cycle (Barnhill & Barnhill, 2002; Brunnicks et al., 1980; Dean, 1976; Reeve et al., 1998).

Few would challenge the positive impact of technological advances on rural life—electricity or air conditioning. TV is viewed in a different light. On the one hand, TV provided information, education and increased awareness of a larger world. But there is a downside. TV meant less time for traditional ways of relating and contributes to a corruption of teaching to and learning of these folkways in children. From this perspective, there is a degree of ambiguity that accompanies new technologies, scientific discoveries, expanding social awareness, and diffusion of urban culture. Many rural folks are feeling overwhelmed as they grapple with their dwindling local heritage, language and speech patterns, music, story-telling, and interpersonal relationships. Taking this argument further, new knowledge and increasing sophistication can be looked upon as "taking away" from the traditional sense of community. On the other hand, TV can help preserve folklore, crafts and music, and other cultural traditions (Gurwitt, 1998; Kessler, 2000).

Widespread social change can be unsettling and can contribute to a counter-reaction or socio-cultural backlash. There are many examples. The "Great Awakenings" of the 18th and 19th centuries were predominantly religious events but served as a backdrop for significant social events—including the American Revolution and the War Between the States. The famous "Scopes Monkey Trial" in Dayton, Tennessee in the early 1920's pitted fundamentalist Christians (including William Jennings Bryan) who were unnerved by growing scientific and social changes of that era against the forces of change and intellectual liberation (including Clarence Darrow and H. L. Menken).

The civil rights movement also reflected the changing face of society and culture.

The reactions of many rural folks (including devoutly "religious" folks) astounded the nation. These occasionally violent reactions tended to reflect the intensity of emotional upheaval or distress to a perceived assault on traditional value systems. The extreme violence and vitriol directed at black and white Americans supporting the civil rights movement is an example. For moderates, "gradualism", "paternalism", and the fears generated by chants of "Black Power" represented less violent reactions but still suggest a need to delay or draw out change. We are seeing this ongoing process of culture change played in a range of more recent "hot-button," divisive issues (Meier, 1969; Klarman, 2003; Cash, 1941).

Conclusions

There is little doubt that geography and population density affect many aspects of service delivery for people living in rural areas. But as we have seen, reliance on measures of population density or geographic distance fails to capture the complex nature of rural America. In fact, social, psychological and cultural factors probably have more to do with the availability and utilization of ID/mental health services than population distribution.

We also need to avoid falling into the trap of thinking that all rural folks have the same values and belief systems. As we have seen in this brief review, the considerable heterogeneity of these regions extends down to even our definition of "rural." Relying on one variable analysis runs the danger of overlooking or homogenizing the significant differences between people who are demographically similar. As noted earlier, there are many rural Americas and any book devoted to service delivery in these settings must account for this heterogeneity.

We need to also consider service delivery in the context of ongoing social-cultural change. In an earlier paper Barnhill & Barnhill (2002) addressed a few of the problems generated when de-institutionalization and the community treatment movements used legal and rhetorical tones that were used a generation earlier during the civil rights struggle. This paper compared the psychosocial responses to reform movements to the larger issues of ongoing culture change. The impact of culture change on rural people struggling to deal with family members with dual diagnosis goes beyond economic, political and legal models and approaches (Magana et al., 2002; Reeve et al., 1998; Anderson, 1995).

In sparsely populated regions, technologies already help manage distance and lack of local services. These innovations permit many clinicians to overcome the scarcity of local expertise and services by using teleconferencing or data sharing via computer linkups. But having technology differs from their integration into the culture of service delivery. It is likely that real progress will not happen until these new technologies and models of service delivery become a part of the local culture.

In closing, the many rural Americas are changing at different rates. Policy makers need to develop ecological models when advocating and instituting changes in the traditional system of care. We need to borrow from evolutionary biologists. Such a model considers the evolution of rural communities within a specific social, cultural, geographic, political, and psychological niche. Institutions such as schools or churches, traditional methods of dealing with problems, and even large residential facilities evolved under similar conditions. From this perspective every community is different and even small changes can produce unexpected outcomes. In short no size fits all and change is unpredictable, but there are solutions out there. We just have to find them.

References

Anderson, R. M. (1995). Revisiting the behavioral model and access to medical care: Does it matter? *Journal of Health and Social Behavior, 36,* 1-10.

Barnhill, S. K. & Barnhill, L. (2002). The role of cultural factors and deinstitutionalization of persons with mental retardation: A view from the rural south. *NADD Bulletin, 5,* 87-92.

Berry, D. (1993). The emerging epidemiology of rural AIDS. *Journal of Rural Health. 9,* 293-304.

Bouras, N., Brooks, D., & Drummond, K. (1994). *Community psychiatric services for people with mental retardation.* London: Cambridge University Press.

Braddock, D., Hemp, R., & Rizzolo, M. (2004). State of the states in developmental disabilities. *Mental Retardation, 42,* 356-370.

Brunnicks, R. H., Thurlow, M., Thurman, K., & Forelli, J. S. (1980). *De-institutionalization and community services* (Vol. XI). New York: Brunner Mazel.

Burnette, D. (2000). Latino grandparents raising children with special needs: Effects on depressive symptomatology. *Journal of Gerontological Social Work, 33*(3), 1-16.

Cash, W. J. (1941). *The mind of the south.* New York: Random House.

Cohn, S. E., Mohr, C. M., & Weber, D. J. (1994). The geography of AIDS: Patterns of urban and rural migration. *Southern Medical Journal, 87,* 599-606.

Dean, A. (1976). *The social system, deviancy, and treatment effects.* New York: Basic Books

Duany, A., Plater-Zybek, E., & Speck, J. (2000). *The rise of sprawl and the decline of the American dream.* New York: North Point Press.

Fox, J., Merwin, E., & Blank, M. (1995). De facto mental health services in the rural south. *Journal of Health Care for the Poor and Underserved, 6,* 434-468.

Fox, J. C., Blank, M., Rovnyak, V. G., & Barnett, R. Y. (2001). Barriers to help for mental disorders in a rural impoverished population. *Community Mental Health Journal, 37,* 421-436.

Greenblatt, M. (1976). *The evolution of the state mental hospital and mental health programs.* New York: Basic Books.

Gurwitt, R. (1998). Keeping the heart in the heartland. *Wilson Quarterly, XXII*(2), 28-36.

Haley, W. E., & Perkins, E. (2004). Current status and future directions in family caregiving and aging people with intellectual disaiblities. *Journal of Policy and Practice in Intellectual Disabilities, 1,* 24-30.

Heller, T., & Factor, A. (1993). Aging family caregivers: Support resources and changes in burden and placement desire. *American Journal on Mental Retardation, 98,* 417-426.

Janicki, M., McCallion, P., Force, L., Bishop, K., & LeProe, P. (1998). Area agency on aging outreach and assistance models for households with older carers of an adult with disability. *Journal of Aging and Social Policy, 10,* 13-36.

Johnson, K. M., Beale, C., Gurwitt, R., & Turner, F. (2000). The rural rebound. *Wilson Quarterly, 22,* 15-42.

Kessler, R. C. (2000). *Sociology and psychiatry.* Philadelphia: Lippincott, Williams, Wilkins.

Klarman, M. J. (2003). *From Jim Crow to civil rights.* New York: Oxford University Press.

Kleinman, A. (1988). *Rethinking psychiatry: From cultural category to personal experience.* New York: Free Press.

Knobbe, C. A., Carey, S., Rhodes, L., & Horner, R. H. (1995). Benefit-cost analysis of community residential versus institutional services for adults with severe mental retardation. *American Journal on Mental Retardation, 99,* 533-541.

Lakin, K. C., Pouty, R., Coucouvanis, B. P. (2004). Fiscal year 2003: Expenditures for Medicaid long term services and supports. *Mental Retardation, 52,* 407-410.

Lewis-Fernandez, R., & Kleinman, A. (1995). Cultural psychiatry: Theoretical, clinical, and research Issues. *Psychiatric Clinics of North America, 18,* 433-448.

Llewellyn, G., Gething, L., Kendig, H., & Cant, R. (2004). Older parent caregivers' engagement with the service system. *American Journal on Mental Retardation, 109,* 379-396.

Magana, S., Seltzer, M., & Kraus, M. W. (2002). Service utilization patterns of adults with intellectual disabilities. *Journal Gerontological Social Work, 37,* 65-86.

Meier, A. (1969). *On the role of Martin Luther King.* Garden City NY: Anchor Books.

Menolascino, F. J. (1994). *Services for people with dual diagnosis in the USA.* London: Cambridge University Press.

National Rural Health Association. (2004). *HIV/AIDS in rural America: Disproportionate impact on minority and multicultural populations.* Kansas City, MO: Author.

Noll, S. (1995). *Feeble-minded in our midst: Institutions for the mentally retarded in the south 1900-1940.* Chapel Hill, NC: University of North Carolina Press.

Ossofsky, G. (1969). *"Come out from among them": Negro migration and settlement.* Garden City, NY: Anchor Books.

Patterson, S., & Friel, L. (2001). Psychological distress, hopelessness, and welfare recipiency. *Women and Health, 32,* 79-99.

Prunchno, R, Patrick, J., & Burant C. J. (1997). African American and white mothers of adults with chronic disabilities: Caregiving burden and satisfaction. *Family Relations, 46,* 335-346.

Prunchno, R. A., & McMullen, W. (2004). Patterns of service utilization by adults with developmental disability: Type of service makes a difference. *American Journal on Mental Retardation, 109,* 362-378.

Reed, J. S. (1974). *The enduring south: Subcultural persistence in mass society.* Chapel Hill, NC: University of North Carolina Press.

Reed, J. S. (1993a). *My tears spoil my aim and other reflections on southern culture.* New York: Harcourt, Brace, & Company.

Reed, J. S. (1993b). *Surveying the south: Studies in regional sociology.* Columbia, MO: University of Missouri Press.

Reeve, A., Aceves, J., Morales, A., Thorne-Lehman, J., & Vickers, J. (1998). Deinstitutionalization: Social policy and social reality. *NADD Bulletin, 1,* 83-88.

Rizzolo, M. C., Hemp, R., Braddock, D., & Pomeranz-Essley, A. (2004). *The state of the states in developmental disabilities.* Washington DC: American Association of Mental Retardation.

Smith, G. C. (1997). Aging families of adults with mental retardation. *American Journal on Mental Retardation, 102,* 13-26.

Turner, F. (1998). The landscape of disturbance. *Wilson Quarterly, XXII*(2), 37-41.

Warner, J. H. (1985). *The idea of southern medical distinctness.* Madison WI: University of Wisconsin Press.

Young, L., & Ashamn, A. (2004). De-institutionalization for older adults with severe mental retardation: Results from Australia. *American Journal on Mental Retardation, 109,* 398-412.

History and Outcome of Various Approaches: Mental Health Services in a Rural Prairie State

Paul D. Kolstoe, PhD, Clinical Director, North Dakota Developmental Center; Steven Hill, MD, Associate Professor, University of North Dakota Medical School; Laurie L. Orvedal, MS, STOP Clinical Coordinator, North Dakota Developmental Center

Introduction

Mental health supports of people with developmental disabilities (DD) are highly contextual, dependent in large part on the types and availability of services. When there is choice, people live where they are likely to survive with their essential needs met.

At the height of "institutionalization" less than 10% of people estimated to have mental retardation were ever served in such settings (Scheerenberger, 1983) including rural states such as North Dakota (Askvig, 2004). The popular myth that such services were extensively used continues to fuel the arguments of advocacy organizations seeking the closure and elimination of such service settings.

Advocacy organizations have been actively critical of segregated residential settings in their unqualified promotion of full integration into generic services (Center on Human Policy at Syracuse University, 2005) since the 1970's. However, it has only been in recent years that the adequacy of generic health care service has become the focus of concern (AAMR National Conference, 2004). Concern about the capacity of generic mental health services has been a long-discussed topic within mental health services for people with DD, as noted by Sovner and Hurley (1986), who cite four issues that confound those giving support. These issues raise concerns about inadequate assessment, misdiagnosis, ineffective (and potentially harmful) treatment, and misdirected residential changes (i.e., jail, hospitalization, institutionalization).

In this chapter we will explore what we have learned about medication use and service delivery for people with DD in a sparse locale. Medication use data will be examined from a state small enough to provide comprehensive information at a time when few researchers are even attempting to examine practices in this area. Further, an overview of the service delivery system's mental health components is described that have evolved in a state physically larger than all of New England with less than 1/20th of the population (1990 Census of Population and Housing, "Population and Housing Unit Counts," CPH-2-1).

North Dakota

The Dakota Territory was separated into North and South Dakota in 1889 as they were admitted into statehood. The Territory first provided mental health services just before the Territorial Capitol moved out of it's first home in Yankton (now South Dakota) to Bismarck (now North Dakota). With the sweeping marble steps that had been imported from Italy as the centerpiece of the building, the Territorial Governor moved the first mental hospital sponsored by the government into the old governor's mansion. Another facility in Jamestown (North Dakota) was also established prior to statehood in 1885 and was the only resource for people needing treatment, safe haven, or community expulsion.

History of Services: 1904 to now

After repeated concerns of the Superintendent at the State Hospital about the divergent needs of people there, the North Dakota legislature established a separate DD service setting at Grafton, North Dakota that opened in May 1904. Education and healthcare were initiated in the first six months it was open, with the growth of the facility steady through the first half of the 20th century. According to Askvig (2004), in the 1930's and 40's the superintendent expressed concerns the facility was grossly undersized. At that time nationally, estimates for the population needing institutionalization (when that was thought to be a GOOD thing) was six to ten times the then current populations. However, at the peak less than 10 percent of those estimated to have mental retardation were ever admitted (Askvig, 2004), which is consistent with national patterns (Scheerenberger, 1983). Reasons that people were admitted to the facility were relatively simple: access to the only educational services available, homelessness/had no one to care for them, healthcare needs exceeding the family's capacity, or behavioral (including mental health) excesses exceeding the local community tolerance (Kolstoe, 1998).

Population shifts in the state continue to follow the general nationwide pattern of movement from rural to urban areas (and out of the state), with 57 percent of the counties in the state with less than five people per square mile and 21 percent with less than three people per square mile. In comparison, Wisconsin's smallest county has 9.5 people per square mile as is true in Vermont – although the next smallest county in Vermont is 38 people per square mile (1990 Census). Simply, distance in the North Central Prairie States is generally discussed in terms of hours or even days rather than in miles.

Deinstitutionalization

Funding lagged behind population growth almost from the beginning of the facility at Grafton. The population peaked in the 1960's in North Dakota and throughout the United States (Scheerenberger, 1987) and began to decrease with the establishment of community education in the 1960's. Despite this gradual decrease in population the conditions at the Grafton facility (and the satellite facility in Dunseith, ND) continued to become more inadequate.

The cultural shift that started with "universal education" rights in the 1960's, became "deinstitutionalization" in the 1970's and 1980's, and extended to the "community imperative" in the 1990's through the present also impacted North Dakota. The state was eventually forced into modernizing services through federal court intervention based upon constitutional issues (ARC v. Olson, 1982; Askvig, 2004).

Under the impetus of the court order to downsize the institutional population to 250 by 1989 (ND ARC v. Olson, 1982), North Dakota completed the deinstitutionalization process below the required levels, met or exceeded the certification and accreditation standards, and the lawsuit was finally settled in 1995. During the time of the lawsuit many changes took place, and a series of measurements were completed during and since that time that are summarized in this chapter.

General Service Delivery System: DD and MI

State Organization

The state is geographically organized into eight approximately equally sized regions, although the regions differ significantly in population. The central office of the human service center is located in the largest city of each region, often with a few satellite offices throughout the region. Although the counties provide many basic social services, the state-owned regional human service centers provide clinical services including substance abuse, mental health services, and developmental disabilities coordination.

It is important to note that all of the regions have private services available to some degree; however, there are few such services beyond the large central community of each region. In particular, two of the eight regions have no inpatient psychiatric center and rely on the central state-operated mental health hospital for acute admission. The state hospital is as much as four hours away on two-lane highways from several points in the regions (even further when considering winter weather conditions).

While there has been a significant effort to provide residential and day services in a handful of small communities, the vast majority of people moving from the state DD facilities relocated in the eight major regional cities.

DD System:

Private providers deliver all developmental disability services. State employee case managers coordinate funding through the regional centers, whose responsibility is to ensure smooth transition across services and life stages. In most aspects, the private providers fulfill most support needs and are seldom dependent upon the state's case managers; however, case management provides system entrance, family support, transition, crisis service coordination and – in the end – is the safety net when there are no other services involved.

Access to psychiatry is through private providers wherever possible (not universal in the eight regions), although the human service centers hire or contract for services to fill gaps. Psychology and behavior analysis has more of a mixed model, with some providers hiring their own behavior analyst while others access such services through the human service center. Healthcare, beyond limited nursing, is exclusively provided by private services in each local or nearby community.

Design and De-reality Within Provider Efforts, Regional Crisis Options

Private providers shift resources, housing, job supports and opportunities, and experienced staff to achieve outcomes for people they serve. They also transition individuals between private providers directly or through coordination at the regional office. Transfers of people between regions also occur when the region's service options are exhausted as determined by the private providers.

Within and between provider resource shifting is used to the extent the system is able to flex, but there are times when the person is deemed dangerous to themselves, others, or to significant property damage. Providers retain the authority to decide if they have the ability to safely serve a person, which means they can also discontinue services if they feel it is necessary. While appeal to the agency's board of directors is always an option for a discharge from services, boards generally uphold administrator actions. This can leave a person homeless.

A few of the largest communities have crisis residential units (CRU's), with various names and configurations, which are operated by or under contract to the human service center. Although this provides some flexibility in a crisis situation, they are generally designed for a person requiring little direct supervision and are extremely challenged to serve people with healthcare issues or more significant personal support needs.

Law Enforcement, Hospitalization and Institutionalization

In 1987-88 a group of psychology and advocacy workers in one region obtained a grant to develop a format for Individual Justice Plans. Originally conceptualized in Nebraska, this strategy is intended to prevent or minimize the behavior occurring again by providing specialized information to the criminal justice system about how to optimize the criminal proceedings and sentencing, along with human service system supports. Although it was published in a manual (Aadland, Afwerke, & Schumacher, 1988), the implementation around the state has had various degrees of success and failure.

In one community the process was embraced relatively well by the service system but only hesitatingly referenced by the courts. In another community there was substantial interest on the part of the police, state's attorney, and court – but little interest from the service system. In 2004 and 2005 the Protection and Advocacy Project sponsored a revision process with resources from a wide range of service and criminal justice specialties to update the manual and to expand the approach for use with people that have mental health (e.g., schizophrenia, bipolar affective disorder) and other cognitive disabilities (e.g., traumatic or acquired brain injury, Asperger Syndrome).

As is true with many states, the record of police, prosecutors, judges, and defense attorneys to recognize and address developmental disabilities is often in the extremes of either failure to ask for assessment or choosing not to prosecute.

Although forensic evaluations are accessible through the Department of Human Services they are inconsistently used (see One Center discussion below).

When a person is removed from their residence to protect themselves, others, or significant property damage it is generally through mental health commitment laws and usually to mental health units in private hospital settings. Statutes were changed in the mid-1990's to require prior authorization of all admissions to the state facilities (mental health and developmental disability) by the regional human service center. The most critical feature of this statute is to permit the local service system to be aware of and intervene in crises that have developed. This has been credited for a significant reduction in the state hospital admissions and increased use of comprehensive community services. When those services are not sufficient, or for acute services for two of the state's regions, state-level services remain available when all other options have systematically been exhausted.

Statewide Safety Net Services: One Center

Vision: One Center – Two Specialized Facilities

The State Hospital serves children and adults with mental health and chemical dependency needs while the Developmental Center serves adults with developmental disabilities with mental health, health, and other support needs. As described above, neither is accessed unless all alternatives have been exhausted. Both facilities have decreased in size since the 1950's (antipsychotics) and 1960's (universal education) peak populations. The state has considered co-location (physical merger) into one site. After multiple legislative reviews – the most recent in 1999 - this was not seen as feasible for a variety of reasons including physical plant, divergence of service formats, and other issues.

In April 2000 the Department of Human Services initiated a merger of the two facilities into a single administrative organization, now often referred to internally as the One Center. Through a series of organizational and personnel moves over the subsequent years, a number of consolidations resulted in reallocations of resources into direct supports. The process uncovered a common mission of the One Center: To support people with disabilities to be viable members of the community when their needs exceed community resources.

For much of the 20th century people were shuttled between the two institutions – often with professional debate as to what the "primary" diagnoses were. Beginning in the late 1980's, the remaining people with mental retardation at the State Hospital were evaluated, and a transition to the Developmental Center was initiated. With the integration of the facilities in 2000, the remaining most-challenging individuals were transitioned with the exception of three whose transfer may be life-threatening.

The most significant impact of the One Center integration was the coordination of state-level crisis support. Previously, providers had the option to use mental health admission to the State Hospital, even when such out-of-community services were not seen as appropriate by the regional or Developmental Center clinical evaluators.

This resulted in a frequent pattern of the person's residential option closing behind them – resulting in being stranded. With organizational integration has come the coordination for maximizing the appropriateness of state level safety net services.

Admission/Transfer/Discharge Coordination - CARES

State-level safety net services in North Dakota must be reserved for people whose needs have exceeded the resources of their local community. For people with developmental disabilities, steps of assessment have to be made at the regional level to determine what other options are available locally. When those resources are exhausted as an option, the regions confer with one another to examine statewide options that may meet the needs of the person. The Developmental Center is involved at this level to become familiar with the situation as it may continue to escalate.

Early in any crisis situation, regions and providers are encouraged to access the consultative outreach program from the ND Developmental Center. The CARES program (Clinical Assistance, Resources, and Evaluation Services) was initiated in 1995 in recognition that providers and regions had been contacting various departments of the Center to obtain support. This support was sometimes disjointed, even contradictory, depending upon who was contacted. The CARES program established a single point of contact from which a team is assembled to address the referral question(s). CARES services have been attractive to support teams as a source of consultation on many issues, but resources have demanded that acceptance into the CARES program be limited to those at risk for losing their community presence.

Several lessons were learned early in the program about the process of consultation. First, NDDC was not designed to provide direct team services so a fully functioning local team must be in place. It is not uncommon that crises have arisen with significant supports missing from the team, and it is an opportunity to work with the local team to add to its membership with the missing pieces. Sometimes the missing piece is just a communication gap between parts of the support network that can also be addressed using assistance, advice, and even, sometimes, mediation.

Another lesson was that the local team often has as much of an answer as anyone will ever obtain; they just need assurance that they are on the right track. Several consultations have amounted to this level of support, which places the NDDC consultants in a "cheer team" role rather than as experts (although the "expert" tag makes cheering more effective). A secondary gain from this is the opportunity of NDDC staff to learn of the creativity, energy, and commitment of the people providing services across the state.

Third, observation by professional staff can be valuable in some situations, but professional observation and communication among direct support staff is often the most productive form of service. We have experienced that sometimes the more credentials the consultant observer has, the more the observation itself becomes tainted by the behavior of the local provider system. When direct contact staff arrive, administrators smile politely and disappear – leaving direct support staff to talk to their peers on a relatively equal, honest level that exposes tremendous amounts of information in very short order. Again, we have often found that the local direct support staff carry significant keys to the answer if their observations are carefully collected.

Finally, no matter how hard the local team works, despite the best brainstorming or the most intense observations, sometimes the person is still unable to be supported to remain in their home community. The goal of ND Developmental Center is to have activated the CARES consultation process for every person before they are referred for admission, but that has not always been practical. Having information prior to admission has been highly useful in maximizing startup of services once at the Center, which in turn can minimize length of stay, and optimize the replication of conditions from home both for the individual's comfort and to plan the transition back home.

Of those admitted to the ND Developmental Center there has been a consistent pattern of heavy psychotropic medication use, generally between three to seven medications being used at the time of admission. By the time of discharge, which can be weeks to years depending upon the complexity of the problems, people tend to be on very few or no psychotropic medications. This may be an effect of the more structured environment (e.g., consistency, stress management, coordination, etc.), a more patient approach to variable separation (e.g., better opportunity for evaluating interventions), or both. While the consulting psychiatrist (second author) serves the facility on a part time basis, the problem solving of multiple medications in the private provider settings is a challenging one. While a given medication may not appear to be effective, provider staff are often very anxious about medication decreases to the existing medication until a new medication has demonstrated effectiveness. When solutions have not been significantly improved, the option of decreasing the previous medication becomes complicated. This has been an observation shared by several psychiatrists around the state.

Medication Utilization In North Dakota: A Longitudinal Examination

The federal court found that North Dakota services violated the constitutional rights of people with developmental disabilities through the inadequate services provided. As a result, the state was ordered to depopulate the institutional setting from over 1,000 people in 1982 to no more than 250 people by 1989. The rapid transition of people from the institutions to community-based services was an opportunity to examine patterns in services.

Trial commenced in January, 1982 and the order was handed down the following May (1983) which required, among other issues, that the state permanently comply with all Title XIX regulations of the Social Security Act (Title XIX - Health Care Finance Administration [HCFA]) by July, 1985 and to comply with all ACMR/DD (now known as The Council) standards by July, 1987 at all facilities where any class member resided (ARC v. Olson, 1982). The standards required included management systems for medication use. The court further required the state to develop community based residential services sufficient to reduce the combined institutional population to 450 by July 1987 and to 250 by July 1989 (since exceeded by reducing to 140). The state has since met these requirements, and the court's involvement ended in May, 1995.

These changes have resulted in the movement of over 700 people from the institution to the community, the closure of the San Haven facility, and compliance by all agencies – as required by the court – with Title XIX and The Council standards, which had been met since the Developmental Center achieved that status in April, 1989 (two years later than was originally ordered by the court).

Under these standards, all psychotropic medications used to modify behaviors, other than seizure-related conditions, must have plans for their use written by the team and reviewed by behavior intervention review and human rights committees (Gardner, 1990). Thus, all individuals with mental retardation in North Dakota receiving psychotropic medications were receiving planning, review, and oversight that have been reported as reducing medication use levels in institutions (Kastner & Walsh, 1994; Rinck, 1998).

North Dakota studies – two longitudinal projects

Larry Burd and his colleagues (Burd, Fisher, Vesely, Williams, Kerbeshian, & Leech, 1991; Burd, Williams, Klug, Fjelstad, Schimke, & Kerbeshian, 1997) worked with the plaintiff's attorney in the ARC v. Olson federal lawsuit to gather service information across the state in 1987 and again in 1993. They gathered information about medication use, in particular, thereby providing rates of use at two points in time. By 1995 the requirements of the lawsuit had been met, and the lead author had the opportunity to examine the archival records of all people residing in the institutions as of 1980 (Kolstoe, 1998). In 1998 the records of each person were reviewed where they resided (regionally or in the institutional setting). The focus was to follow the medication use patterns prior to the initiation of the lawsuit in 1980, in 1989 when the regulatory and population levels of the lawsuit were fully achieved, and then again in 1995 following several years of stability of standards implementation which led to closing the court's need for oversight.

Community medication use levels

Medication in the community context was first addressed by Gowdey, Zarfas, and Phipps (1987) in Ontario, Canada, but they included all psychoactive medications in their study (i.e., antiepileptic in addition to neuroleptic, anxiolytic, antidepressant, etc.) to arrive at the overall medication rate of 40% for people with mental retardation who lived in community group homes. This is inconsistent with the usual institutional reporting methods, where seizure medications were not typically counted together with other psychoactives (Poindexter, 1989; Rivinus, 1980). However, Gowdy et al. did report rates on the use of the individual classes of medications: 14%, neuroleptics; 5%, sedative/hypnotics; 3%, antidepressants; and 1%, antimanic. This reflected an overall rate of approximately 23% of people on psychotropic medications other than seizure medications.

Buck and Sprague (1989) used a slightly different methodology to measure psychotropic medications by examining the Medicaid billing patterns for community Medicaid funded facilities in the communities of Illinois. They used pharmacy billing information to determine medications given to individuals included in the study, although they cautioned that it did not represent all individuals with mental retardation living in the community. Their findings were specific to traditional psychoactive medications as they did not count any antiepileptic medications, establishing the rate of 28.9% of the target population receiving such medications. Although the authors found this rate to be comparable with nursing home patients without mental retardation in facilities funded in the same manner, the use of neuroleptic medications was somewhat higher; 88% of people with mental retardation on psychotropic medications received neuroleptics as opposed to 74% of nursing home patients in that time (mid-1980's).

It is important to note that the names of these different classes of medications have reflected, to a large extent, the intended condition for which they are commonly used (e.g., anti-depressant for depression, anxiolytic for anxiety); however, the use is not restricted by such classification (Bates, Smeltzer, & Arnoczky, 1986). For people with mental retardation there has been significant use of medication with disorders outside of the original class for which it was named, such as the relatively common practice to use antiepileptic medications for mood disorders (Burd et al., 1991).

North Dakota medication use levels

Burd, Fisher et al. (1991) conducted their survey of all group homes in North Dakota in 1988 and again in 1993 (Burd, Williams et al., 1997) in order to comprehensively establish the rate of medication use. They received a 97% and 100%, return rate, respectively, that revealed a psychotropic medication prevalence rate of 37% in 1988 and 38% in 1993. The North Dakota researchers (Burd, Fisher et al., 1991; Burd, Williams et al., 1997) used the same procedures as Gowdey et al. (1987) in that their methodology included antiepileptic medications in the data collection. The North Dakota research teams were attempting to incorporate the fact that antiepileptic medications were increasingly being used to treat non-seizure related disorders such as behavioral problems and some psychiatric symptoms. When eliminating anti-epileptic medications (note, NOT based on presence of a seizure disorder), the prevalence rate of medication use drops to 18% in 1988 and 20% in 1993. These rates (37%:18% and 38%:20%) are relatively similar to that found by Gowdey et al. (40%:23%).

Community rates of medication use, from what little information is available, appear to be in the range of 18% to 40% depending upon the medications examined and the population sampled. In contrast, PRF levels were historically described as between 25% and 64% depending upon when data were collected, contemporanious standards, and medications chosen for review. In several more recent reports (Briggs, 1989; Findholt & Emmett, 1990; Poindexter, 1989; Rinck, 1998; Stone, Alvarez, Ellman, Horn, & White, 1989; Zaharia, 1986) investigators report rates in the 10% to 24% range which is somewhat lower than previous PRF rates and available community rates.

Institutional medication levels

By following those people originally residing in the institution later in their life, the majority of whom moved to community settings, a more direct examination of medication use patterns across settings is performed. In that the same service providers were involved in both studies, there is the opportunity to learn more about the experiences with medications of the people served in North Dakota.

Prevalence data on medication use in institutions has historically been well documented to be at levels considered excessive. Rivinus (1980) conducted a systematic search of the literature, reviewing 166 studies from the 1960's through the 1980's regarding the use of medications on people with mental retardation. He noted a series of studies which were completed on medication use rates in public facilities across the United States. These surveys reported institutional psychotropic drug use rates to generally be between 51% and 64%. Lipman (1970) surveyed 109 facilities on medication use and found that they averaged 51%.

Rivinus (1980) noted one state where one facility was large and the other was small, each had a highly similar rate of 50% of the population receiving psychotropic medications. In another case, a relatively stable average of 47% of the people served across five facilities in eastern Canada were receiving neuroleptic medications. As a further example in a state with two facilities, with an important twist, 53% of the people received psychotropic drugs in one and 25% in the other, despite being of comparable size and population type.

Rivinus also reported a survey of the facility in which he was working and noted the incidence of neuroleptics use – alone – to be 57% prior to the availability of regular psychiatric consultation. Further, a rate of polypharmacy was noted in 27% of the people. After four years of regular psychiatric consultation the neuroleptic drug use was reduced to 23% and polypharmacy was eliminated completely. Four conclusions from these surveys were identified (1980, p. 198):

1. Psychotropic agents have come into widespread, poorly controlled, and poorly reviewed use in institutions for mentally retarded persons.
2. Polypharmacy is practiced widely in institutions.
3. The use of drugs is often the measure of the lack of alternative approaches to unacceptable behavior and programmatic shortcomings in most institutions for retarded persons.
4. Psychotropic agents can effectively be part of the responsible treatment and

habilitative programs for some institutionalized retarded persons.

He went on to point out that by 1980 "studies of the effect of psychotropic agents on the functioning of noninstitutionalized retarded [sic] patients are rare or inconclusive; there is a need for such studies" (p. 199).

Following up on Rivinus' article, Aman and Singh (1986) reviewed nine new research reports on medication use rates in institutions. They observed no real change in psychotropic drug use rates among public residential facilities. While finding that between 40 and 50% of institutional residents could be expected to be receiving psychotropic medication at any given time, they conclude that people with mental retardation are probably among the most medicated people in society.

Longitudinal institutionalized cohort

Prior to the onset of the ARC v. Olson lawsuit, the medication levels at the North Dakota institutions (at Grafton and Dunseith) had not been questioned by lawsuit investigation or the implementation of federal service standards. The institutional rates prior to the implementation of standards imposed either by lawsuit investigation or court requirement were measured from the archived files with coding respect to the use of the antiepileptic medications.

Medication use levels at each time frame (1980, 1989, and 1995) were collected in terms of their apparent function according to the orders of the time. Four categories were established: psychoactive medications included antiepileptic and traditional psychiatric medications, psychiatric medications excluded those antiepileptics used for seizure management, neuroleptics consisted of the antipsychotics (including atypicals), and seizure medications reflect antiepileptics used for seizure management.

Medication use levels as of January 1, 1980 are reflected in Figure 1. Comparison with similar settings from similar institutional eras finds these levels within the norm of institutional settings at 55.4 percent of all psychoactive medications, compared to rates mentioned earlier of 51 to 64 percent (Lipman, 1970).

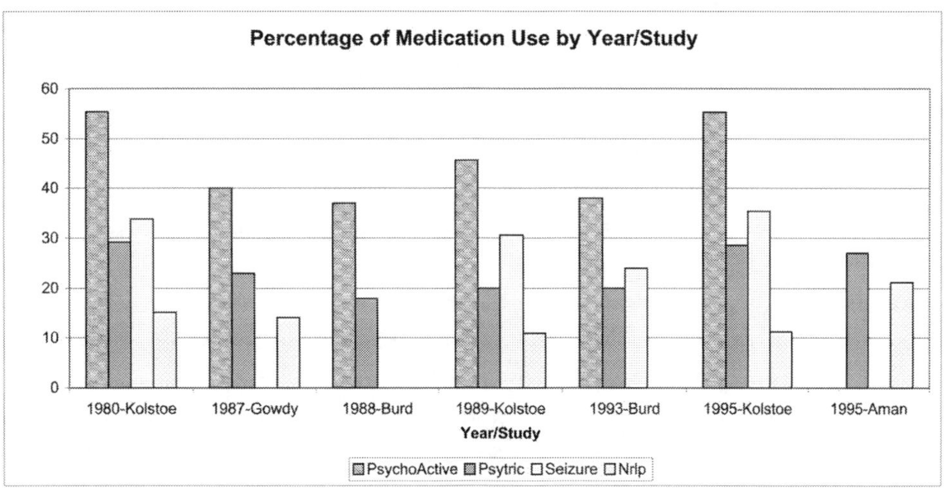

Although it is clear those people remaining in the institution experienced an overall decrease in medication use across all categories, the same was true of the general population of people originally in the institution in 1980. However, the fact that proportions of every group returned to near base-line levels is a rather astonishing finding. The important exception to this rebound is the Neuroleptic class of medications, which dropped by about one-third in their use (15.1% to 10.1%) and remained there in 1995 (11.2%).

At least 15 of those institutionalized in 1995 were known to have been placed into the community and returned to the Center, in some cases with several attempts. Of very positive note, only two of those people were returned during the 1989 to 1995 time period. Of the individuals remaining at the Center in the late 1990's, about one-third of the 1995 facility population had never been admitted to the Center until this admission.

The individuals residing in the community generally do not require a higher use of medications in comparison with those "left behind" in the institution. To the contrary, individuals in the institution are given psychoactive medications at a higher rate than the community counterparts (58.4% to 39.7%), but this is primarily as a result of seizure medication use rates (40.8% to 25.6%). This was not the case for either Psychiatric Use (24% and 18%) medications or the subset Neuroleptics (10.9% and 10.4%). Both groups sustain their decrease in Neuroleptics through 1995 (10.9% to 11.2%), but the general return towards 1980 proportions in medications use is pervasive across all other categories despite setting.

Conclusions

Mental/behavioral health services in North Dakota have evolved through the deinstitutionalization process to successfully serve most citizens in their home community. The institutional settings (Developmental Center and State Hospital) have been integrated to insure that people are supported in the most appropriate state level service setting to their needs – but only after all community alternatives have been exhausted.

Very few people with mental retardation in North Dakota require state-level services (140 of over 3,000 on caseload – 4.7 percent), and those who experience challenges to remaining in their home community have local crisis support options, service alternatives, and CARES consulting to support them. However, these services are of limited size and primarily in population centers that may be significant distance from their preferred community.

Medication use in North Dakota reflected the socio-cultural decrease of the "anti-medication" movement of the 1980's, and this was even reflected in the use of seizure medications. Although overuse of medication was cited as a concern about institutional services at the time of the lawsuit, the pre-lawsuit medication use rates returned by 1995 within the same cohort of people – whether they remained in the facility or moved to the community. In addition, community-based service measurements of medication use rates – when compared to those of the institutional/deinstitutionalized population cohort – reflected similar levels and patterns between the groups (who had many of the same people in both groups).

If institutional use of medications was excessive prior to the lawsuit in North Dakota, then the levels of medication use have returned to the population of people with mental retardation served in the community settings. While medications no longer appear to have the negative stigma attached to their use, and there is little current concern about over medication among people with MR/DD, there is significant room for further investigation in this area now that services are "genericised" and distributed around the state/private providers.

While there is great debate about the necessity of institutional settings, North Dakota community service providers continue to find limits to their capacity to serve everyone needing support. Safeguards designed to prevent institutionalization into either the mental health or the developmental disabilities system has been effective at preventing wholesale escalation of state-level services, and yet there continues to be a stable level of population referred to that level of service. While rural settings continue to try to develop crisis service capacity, it is generally limited to larger urban centers. Is an institution specializing in services to people with developmental disabilities a necessary component of the range of services to people in a rural state like North Dakota? The philosophical answer remains unclear but at present the practical response currently reflects that there continues to be a need for a setting with well-coordinated professional expertise, socio-behavioral structure, and more immediate resource reallocation than can currently be delivered in private services in this state. A more pertinent question becomes whether those services can be generated across such a rural state, or would they simply be re-created in a few urban settings marginally closer to the individual's actual home community?

References

Aadland, J. Afwerke, P., & Schumacher, K. (1988). *Individual justice planning: A training manual.* State of North Dakota.

AAMR National Conference. (2004, June). *Community health supports: Facing the challenge,* Philadelphia, PA.

Aman, M. G. & Singh, N. N. (1986). A critical appraisal of recently drug research in mental retardation: The Coldwater studies. *Journal of Mental Deficiency Research, 30,* 203-216.

ARC v. Olson, 713 F. 2d 1384 (D.C.N.D. 1982).

Askvig, B. A. (2004). *One hundred years: The history and chronology of the North Dakota Developmental Center.* Minot, N.D. : North American Heritage Press.

Bates, W. J., Smeltzer, D. J., & Arnoczky, S. M. (1986). Appropriate and inappropriate use of psychotherapeutic medications for institutionalized mentally retarded persons. *American Journal on Mental Deficiency, 90,* 363-370.

Briggs, R. (1989). Monitoring and evaluating psychotropic drug use for persons with mental retardation: A follow-up report. *American Journal on Mental Retardation, 93,* 633-

639.

Buck, J. A., & Sprague, R. L. (1989). Psychotropic medication of mentally retarded residents in community long-term care facilities. *American Journal on Mental Retardation, 93,* 618-623.

Burd, L., Fisher, W., Vesely, B. N., Williams, M., Kerbeshian, J., & Leech, C. (1991). Prevalence of psychoactive drug use among North Dakota group home residents. *American Journal on Mental Retardation, 96,* 119-126.

Burd, L., Williams, M., Klug, M. G., Fjelstad, K., Schimke, A., & Kerbeshian, J. (1997). Prevalence of psychotropic and anticonvulsant drug use among North Dakota group home residents. *Journal of Intellectual Disability Research, 41,* 488-494.

Findholt, N. E. & Emmett, C. G. (1990). Impact of interdisciplinary team review on psychotropic drug use with persons who have mental retardation. *Mental Retardation, 28,* 41-46.

Gardner, J. F. (1990). Application of behavior intervention standards for individual with a developmental disability and a mental health diagnosis. *ACDD Accreditation Update Newsletter, 7 (2),* 4.

Gowdey, C. W., Zarfas, D. E., & Phipps, S. (1987). Audit of psychoactive drug prescriptions in group homes. *Mental Retardation, 25,* 331-334.

Kastner, T. A. & Walsh, K. (1994). Exchange of views on psychotropic drug review: Interdisciplinary team review of psychotropic drug use in community settings. *Mental Retardation, 32,* 243-245.

Kolstoe, P. D. (1998). Deinstitutionalization effects on medication use for people with mental retardation. University of North Dakota Dissertation.

Lipman, R. S. (1970). The use of pharmacological agents in residential facilities for the retarded. In F. J. Menoliscino (Ed.), *Psychiatric approaches to mental retardation.* (pp. 387-398). New York: Basic Books.

Poindexter, A. R. (1989). Psychotropic drug patterns in a large ICF/MR facility: A ten-year experience. *American Journal on Mental Retardation, 93,* 624-626.

Rinck, C. (1998). Epidemiology and psychoactive medication. In S. Reiss & M. G. Aman (Eds.), *Psychotropic medications and developmental disabilities: The International Consensus handbook* (pp. 31-44). Columbus, OH: The Ohio State University Nisonger Center.

Rivinus, T. (1980). Psychopharmacology and the mentally retarded patient. In L. S. Szymanski & P. E. Tanguay (Eds.), *Emotional disorders of mentally retarded persons: Assessment, treatment, and consultation* (pp. 195-221). Baltimore, MD: University Park Press.

Scheerenberger, R. C. (1983*). A history of mental retardation.* Baltimore, MD: Paul H. Brookes Publishing Co.

Scheerenberger, R. C. (1987*). A_history of mental retardation: A quarter century of promise.* Baltimore, MD: Paul H. Brookes Publishing Co.

Sovner, R. & Hurley, A. D. (1986). Four factors affecting the diagnosis of psychiatric disorders in mentally retarded persons. *Psychiatric Aspects of Mental Retardation Reviews, 5,* 46-48.

Stone, R. K., Alvarez, W. F., Ellman, G., Hom, A. C., & White, J. F. (1989). Prevalence and prediction of psychotropic drug use in California developmental centers. *American Journal on Mental Retardation, 93,* 627-632.

The Community Imperative (n.d.) Retrieved May, 2005 from http://thechp.syr.edu/community_imperitive.html

1990 Census of Population and Housing, "Population and Housing Unit Counts," CPH-2-1.

Retrieved on May 25, 2005 from http://quickfacts.census.gov/qfd/states/00000.html

Zaharia, E. S. (1986). Reducing reliance on psychotropic drugs. *Superintendents' Digest - NASPRFMR, 5,* 11-13. (National Association of Superintendents of Public Residential Facilities for Mental Retardation).

Coming Home on the Range: Changing Profiles of the People Served and the Provision of Their Community and Institutional Services in Rural Wyoming, 1988-2004

Ken B. Heinlein, Wyoming Institute for Disabilities, UCEDD, University of Wyoming; David J. Heath, Jon Fortune, Wyoming Developmental Disabilities Division, Wyoming Department of Health; Robert M. Lynch, University of Northern Colorado, Kenneth W. Monfort College of Business; Barbara Fortune, Family Practice Center, University of Wyoming

For adults with developmental disabilities, the community programs of the early 21st Century significantly differ from what they were when they emerged in the 1960s. Staffing, funding, regulations, and expectations are greater. With the expansion of Medicaid waivers, state funding and regulations have been displaced by federal funds and regulations, and with that the locus of control for administrative decisions has shifted. Professionally trained staff have replaced volunteers. Expectations have been broadened as parents and professionals, under the influence of such visionaries as Wolfensberger (1972), sought greater participation for persons with mental retardation. The development of community alternatives both influenced and was influenced by the efforts to downsize state residential institutions. By 1970 the national census of persons served in institutions was declining (Bassuk & Gerson, 1978; Lakin, Bruininks, & Sigford, 1981; Lakin, Prouty, Blake, & Mangan, 1993), a trend which continues.

States with large populations like California and New York (Jacobson, Sersen, & Schwartz, 1984) have published statewide descriptions. We describe a service population and the challenges and changes encountered in providing services to persons with developmental disabilities in Wyoming, a predominantly rural state.

Structural Changes

In Wyoming, the development of community programs for persons with mental retardation and other developmental disabilities was similar to the national trend, though delayed about a decade. Associations of parents initiated most programs for developmentally disabled persons in the 1970s. These early programs were often staffed by volunteers. The first group homes, about 25 financed by the Department of Housing and Urban Development (HUD), emerged in the late 1970s and early 1980s. Archie McCulla, a retired national HUD administrator who settled in the state, helped Wyoming develop some of the first housing for adults with developmental disabilities starting with a project in Evansville in the late 1970s. The regional non-profit service organizations, which presently provide services to about 1995 adults, were formed by the middle of the 1980s. Trained staff replaced volunteers and voluntary donations were replaced first by Title 20 funds in the 1970s and later by state general funds in fiscal year 1980. In the early 1990s, Medicaid home and community-based waiver funds became and remain the primary source of funding.

The increase in government support led to increased government regulations, involvement, and expectations. Throughout the 1980s, Wyoming had one state administrator to oversee the nine regional adult DD service providers and one for the 14 regional DD preschool service providers. An additional person was added after P.L. 99-457 authorized infant and toddler services through what was then called Part H of the Education for All Handicapped Children Act, now called Part C of the Individuals with Disabilities Education Act. The Developmental Disabilities Division now has 39 people in the state office, including field office staff.

By 2005, the thirty pages of rules for the selection of DD adult, DD preschool, mental health, and substance abuse service providers had been replaced with a 33 page set of regulations for adult DD waiver providers. Presently, there are about 950 waiver service providers, and a program of $78.2 million for home and community based services for people with developmental disabilities

Concurrent with the increase in government support and increase in community alternatives, the number of persons served at Wyoming's only institution, the State Training School, decreased. The Training School reached its peak population of 742 residents in 1972 and slowly declined until tight budgets in the late 1980s stalled the process. The filing of a lawsuit (Weston, et al. v. WSTS, et al., C90-0004) in 1990 established, and the subsequent Settlement Agreement in 1996 maintained, specific census ceilings that led to sharply reducing the Training School's population. Between 1988 and 2004, Wyoming reduced its enrollment at the Training School from 389 to 93 residents. Most of the reduction occurred as a result of the requirements of the Settlement Agreement and were funded through the state's Medicaid adult and child home and community-based waivers.

Implementing Community Alternatives

The development of Wyoming's community alternatives faced the same challenges of service availability and assurances of quality as other states, but on a different demographic stage. Wyoming's 506,529 citizens occupy 97,812 square miles. It is the least populous of the 50 United States. Wyoming has seven towns with 8,900 to 20,000 people, and only three greater than that. One has 27,204, another has 49,644 and the capital city, Cheyenne, is the largest with 54,374. Towns are frequently separated by 100 miles. Access to emergency medical care is often provided by helicopter, and many parts of the state are classified as health care manpower shortage areas. Equally short are the persons trained to work with persons who have developmental disabilities. Wyoming is ranked 45th with 202 non-federal physicians per 100,000 persons and 37th with 708 nurses per 100,000 persons (Bitner, 2004).

A rural state presents special challenges for community placements and raises the question if people with developmental disabilities can live successfully and find the support they need in small frontier towns after leaving the care of an institution. The challenge in Wyoming posed by rapid deinstitutionalization was heightened by several factors. The state did not have an intermediate care facility for the mentally retarded (ICF/MR) prior to 1990 nor a home and community-based waiver prior to 1991. The community provider organizations offered a limited array of services, in keeping with limited state support.

Two additional problems in rural service provision were the difficulties caused by little or no public transportation and adverse climate due in part to the wind and high altitude of the state, an average elevation of about 6,700 feet above sea level, second only to Colorado. The climate is challenging and distances between cities and towns are great. During the winter there are frequent periods when the winds reach 35 miles per hour with gusts to 55 miles per hour. Prevailing winds sculpt the trees in characteristic patterns. Casper for example, a city located near the center of the state, has average winds of 13 miles per hour with highs at 81 miles per hour (World Almanac, 2005). Each year the average consumer service location has an average of five blizzards resulting from at least five inches of snow, low temperatures and high winds. The climate, distances, and low population densities limit service choice for individuals with developmental disabilities.

The waivers were a fortunate and timely coincidence for the further development of community services, because they greatly increased the amount of money available to purchase services and increased the array of services. This allowed community providers to shape services by individually writing plans of care and tailoring services to support the people served. Lakin (2004) ranked Wyoming 14th in the nation with more than 79.6% of total spending allocated to community services. Wyoming was the 24th state with cost per participant spending on adult and child home and community-based waivers and 26th in combined home and community based waiver and ICF/MR spending (Lakin, 2004).

What follows is a pair of cross sectional analyses of the changing state system for services to people with developmental disabilities. The cross sections were taken in 1988 and 2004, using the Inventory for Client and Agency Planning (ICAP), (Bruninks, Hill, Weatherman, & Woodcock, 1986). The Wyoming Division of Developmental Disabilities' (Division) data set includes all individuals receiving services funded by the Division whether served in the community or institutional programs. Data were collected in 1988 and 2004, sixteen years between which a significant and rapid depopulation of the state institution occurred.

ICAP Studies

Wyoming selected the Inventory for Client and Agency Planning (ICAP) because prior research provided initial support for its use. Wikoff (1989) indicated the ICAP was developed by "state-of-the-art" psychometric techniques and should be used to aid in screening, monitoring, managing, planning and evaluating services for persons who have handicaps, disabilities or are elderly. Johnson (1989) suggested its use as a preliminary screening device and as a research criterion measure for investigations into the global effects of short- and long-term training programs. Thurlow (1989) provides an example in a study reporting positive employment outcomes for special education students who have transitioned to work in the community. Other studies provided evidence for criterion related validity of measures of adaptive and maladaptive behavior and suggested that such skills provide an important contribution to community adaptation and to program and decision making for individuals (Walker & Prazak, 1989; Haugen, 1990; McGrew, Bruininks, & Thurlow, 1992; DeStefano, 1992).

McGrew, Ittenbach, Bruininks, and Hill (1991) factor analyzed data to provide information on the structure of maladaptive behavior relative to age and degree of mental retardation. The study considered 8,255 persons with mild to profound mental retardation, ranging in age from birth to 98 years of age. Across samples, as many as six different dimensions were identified, ranging from two principal factors for children to four factors for older adults, indicating that the structure of maladaptive behavior is influenced by age and level of mental retardation. In 1993, Chen, Bruininks, Lakin, and Hayden, using items originating from the ICAP to measure problem behavior, determined that personal competencies were least important in distinguishing between people living in small group homes or small foster homes. Primary differences emerged in factors assessing the extent of community participation, family relationships, and recreation/leisure integration.

Deinstitutionalization Studies

Many positive results from deinstitutionalization are noted in the literature from around the world in the early portion of this century. Spreat and Conroy (2002) found that family contact increased prior to the move to the community and these increased levels of contact were maintained for as long as four years. Results from Australia reported by Young and Ashman (2004) suggest that positive results were evident for older adults with severe mental retardation. Research by Young, Ashman, Sigafoos, and Grevell (2001) in Queensland showed improvements in adaptive functioning, life circumstances, and increased opportunities for choice-making following relocation to the community but no significant change in maladaptive behavior. Emerson (2004) reports that 93% of British individuals who moved out of National Health Service long-stay hospital "beds" to the community from 1976 to 2002 enjoyed a range of benefits, including increases in satisfaction, social inclusion, engagement, and support, but there appears to be little impact on levels of challenging behavior. Canadian results reported by Quinsey, Book, and Skilling (2004) suggest the deinstitutionalization of men with intellectual disabilities who have been institutionalized may be dangerous. Some are considered to be at high risk for the commission of serious antisocial acts or sexual offending. It was recommended that measures of dynamic risk from staff ratings are worth developing and evaluating. Jahoda and Markova (2004) followed ten people with intellectual disabilities who wrestled with social stigma as they moved to community care in Scotland Results from the United Kingdom and Wales by Perry and Felce (2003) suggest that in 47 small scale, community-based residential settings better life outcomes tended to be significantly correlated with the ability of the resident. Kim, Larson, and Lakin (2001) included the Wyoming and 37 other longitudinal studies from 1980 to 1999 that described robust and consistent positive results from the movement of people from residential institutions to their home communities during the last century.

For Wyoming, Fortune, Heinlein, and Fortune (1995) described a six-year (1988 to 1994) change in distribution of ICAP service scores and characteristics of the populations of those served in Wyoming's institution and communities as the deinstitutionalization process was underway. By the end of 2004, the census of all persons served in community or institutional settings was updated. The 1988 and 2004 censuses using the ICAP provide snapshots of the changes in the community and the residential institutional populations during the sixteen-year period. The designated populations and services changed as Wyoming focused on and assisted people with developmental disabilities in their move to the communities of the Cowboy State. From the Division's databases, the writers were able to identify changes and challenges in service provision in 1988 and 2004.

Before we begin to discuss the results of these two census point, we would like to discuss the ICAP in detail.

ICAP Scoring

The Division uses the Inventory for Client and Agency Planning (ICAP) (Bruininks, Hill, Weatherman, & Woodcock, 1986) to assess the adaptive functioning, problem behavior, functional characteristics, and service needs of clients with developmental disabilities. Leal (1992) identified that the ICAP was statistically related to the Scales of Independent Behavior (SIB) and the Woodcock-Johnson Psycho-Educational Battery. The ICAP measures adaptive behavior in four domains—social and communication, personal living, community living, and motor. The problem behavior scale measures maladaptive behavior in three areas—internalized, externalized, and asocial. The ICAP maladaptive score ranges from 0 to -74 with a standard deviation of -10. For example, no maladaptive problems would be indicated by a score of zero and serious maladaptive behavior problems would be represented by increasingly larger negative numbers such as -35. The broad independence scores range from 306 to 554.

The ICAP service score is the weighted average of the adaptive (.7) and maladaptive (.3) score and ranges from 0 to 100. The ICAP service level ranges from 1 to 9. Persons receiving an ICAP level 1 service score can be expected to require total care and intensive supervision and a level 9 represents total independence. Levels 4 through 6 identify supervised intermediate care and levels 7 through 9 indicate that limited supervision is likely to be required. The ICAP was developed recognizing that adaptive and problem behaviors interact and that neither score alone is sufficient to predict the level of service required. The service needs section of the ICAP combines adaptive behavior and problem behavior scores to yield an overall measure (called the service score) of the individual's need for care, support, supervision, and training. The test-retest and interrater reliabilities are in the .8 to .9 range (Bruininks, Woodcock, Hill & Weatherman, 1985).

The Division has used the Inventory for Client and Agency Planning (ICAP) in describing people served and their selection of services. The ICAP has been used by 26 other states such as Montana, New Mexico, South Dakota, and Utah as a convenient database. It can compile information at the local, regional or state level and provides easily operated computer software for generating individual client reports or group profile summaries. The ICAP results are sometimes used for determining state funding levels for individuals such as in Utah's adult with developmental disabilities home and community-based waiver or New Mexico's state funding. The ICAP may be of some value (though it is best supplemented with additional measures) in the difficult job of matching financial resources to the individual level of need of the people served. For example, Campbell et al. (2005) describe a convincing individual budget model using shared ICAP statewide data for the three states of Montana, South Dakota, and Wyoming. There are a number of instruments other than the ICAP in use in other states, such as The Client Development Evaluation Report, Minnesota ICF/MR Client Assessment Form, Wisconsin Community Options Program Functional Screen, and the Revised Adaptive Behavior Scale. In 1986, Brown et al. developed The Developmental Disabilities Profile for New York that provides assessments in adaptive, maladaptive, and health areas while having value in determining cost. This brief and easy to use instrument has been used with some success by the state of Kansas (Chapin, 1991) and been explored in Alabama, Delaware, and New Jersey. The Supports Intensity Scale (SIS) emerged in 2004 published by the American Association on Mental Retardation (Thompson et al.) focusing on the pattern and intensity of supports needed to enable a person to participate in valued settings and activities. This scale provides a nice counterpoint for overall system redesign, especially the individual planning process.

Additional research is needed to identify and document the strengths and weaknesses of the ICAP instrument and other instruments as they are used to describe basic characteristics of individuals with developmental disabilities who transition from residential institutions in rural areas. There are aspects of this written description of clients that could benefit from supplemental measures. For example, it is true that the ICAP does not have strong sections to document social integration/barriers, medical complications, physical disabilities, leisure and recreation, or unlawful behavior. Additionally, as is the case with most measures of maladaptive behavior, the ICAP behavior section provides only a rough profile at best of the nature or intensity of the behavior. The value of descriptions of groups of people served offered by this effort does not provide an assessment of the individual's living circumstances. An absence of demonstrated skills (such as might be apparent for someone living in an institution) or the demonstration of challenging behavior might have little to do with individual capacity. Instead, environmental factors like poorly trained staff or lack of opportunity may have an enormous influence on individual scores. Finally, given the field of developmental disabilities' current emphasis on inclusion, combined with the paradox of increasingly common waiting lists, this description using the ICAP and most other similar instruments does not offer particular insight into the individual's capacity for participating in or contributing to his or her community. As a result, a unitary reliance on the ICAP as a means for collecting information, would provide only a narrow, though useful and basic, profile of an individual's adaptation and lifestyle.

Results

In 1988, Wyoming served 875 individuals in the Training School and its community-based system of services for individuals with developmental disabilities. By 2004, that number had increased to 1,845, although it would be misleading to imply that all of the original 875 persons were included in the 1,845 The composition of the 2004 group changed from 1988 through transfers to and from other states, independent placements, withdrawals from services, and deaths, as well as an influx of students aging out of special education services. Of the 875 who were receiving services in 1988, more than half (455) were still receiving services in 2004. The size of population served in 2004 was nearly double that in 1988. As the data will show, the community developed greater capacity to serve a wide range of individuals challenged by developmental disabilities and other secondary disorders.

Both census points are demographically similar to the population of Wyoming as measured by the 2000 Census. About 6.4% were of Hispanic origin of any race, 92.1% white, 2.3% American Indian, .8% black, .6% Asian, and 2.5% from other races. All of the individuals from both groups understood English except ten who understood Spanish and twelve who understood another language like Native American dialects. The median age in Wyoming for the general population is 32 years of age while the community group averaged 42 years of age and the institutional group averaged 52 years of age.

The 1988 and 2004 statewide populations distributions were similar with some decrease as indicated in Table 1.

The average ICAP service score was 56 with a *SD* of 27 in 1988, 52 in 2004. In other words, the ICAP results suggest the average client in the system needed a moderate level of supervision. The broad independence score decreased 68 points and the average age decreased by seven years during the interval, largely an artifact of the addition of the children's waiver in 1994.

Maladaptive behavior scores also declined. The average in 1988 was -14 and in 2004 the average was -19. In 1988 and in 2004, 8% of the people served face the dual challenges posed by developmental disabilities and serious mental health challenges like depression and schizophrenia. This is reflected in the overall maladaptive score of -19 for the entire 2004 group.

What is different is the shift to community-based services for many individuals who were once at the Training School and the expansion of community services for many more children and adults. In 1988, before Wyoming had an ICF/MR or waivers, the 389 persons were served by the Training School and 486 persons served by the adult community service providers. By 2004 the census at the Training School decreased to 93 and the community based programs increased to 1,845 individuals.

Table 1
ICAP Results in 1988 and 2004

	1988		2004	
	Mean	Range	Mean	Range
Statewide				
Broad Independence	459	306-554	391	306-535
Maladaptive	-14	-63 to 0	-19	-51 to 0
Service Score	56	1-99	52	1-92
Age	37	3-87	30	8-91
N =	875		1,845	
Community				
Broad Independence	495	06-554	440	306-535
Maladaptive	-9	-46 to 0	-8	-51 to 0
Service Score	74	15-99	52	1-92
Age	35	16-70	42	1-91
N =	486		1,752	
Institution				
Broad Independence	412	306-519	384	306-471
Maladaptive	-20	-63 to 0	-6	-30 to 0
Service Score	33	1-88	32	13-71
Age	41	3-87	52	20-86
N =	389		93	

In 1988, the Training School residents had an average service score of 33 or level 3 with a *SD* of 20, virtually unchanged at 32, level 3 in 2004. During the same interval, the average broad independence score decreased from 412 to 384. However the average maladaptive index score -20 in 1988 increased to -6 in 2004. The Training School, the state's centralized ICF/MR, was still serving many of the individuals with the most severe challenges, especially in the medical and sometimes behavioral area, and had an aging population age as indicated by an increase in the average age from 41 in 1988 to 52 in 2004.

Figure 1

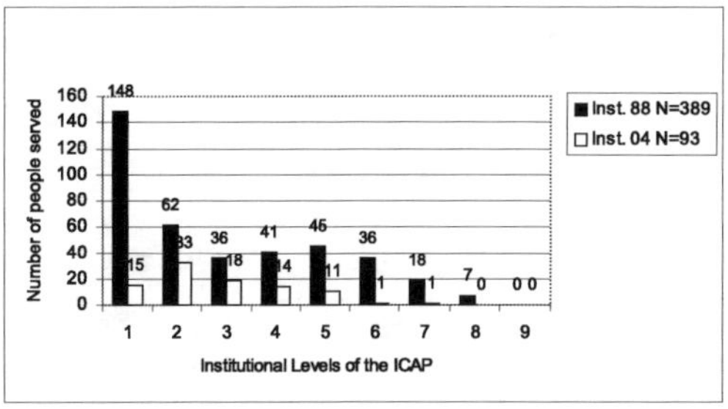

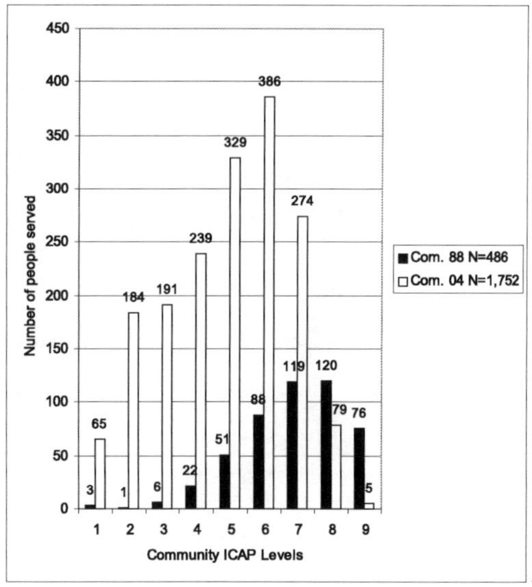

An examination of Figure 1 shows that fewer people were served at the Training School at all ICAP levels in 2004 than in 1988. The change in the distribution was the result of mortality, movement to community programs, and, in the case of the older persons served at WSTS, nursing home placements. The change is most dramatic at level 1, with a 96% decrease in the number of persons served, level 2 reduced to half the former people, and in the mid-range, levels 4-6, with reductions of 88%. The number of individuals in all of the ICAP levels of need have increased for individuals served in the community, showing the movement of Wyoming citizens with developmental disabilities with a wide range of challenges to the community and the expansion of services to children through the Children's Waiver. The most dramatic increases for the community service providers are in levels 1-3, which are characterized by individuals who require total or extensive care. The number of individuals served in the community at levels 4 increased almost 11-fold. The community developed the ability to serve many more people in the level 5-7 range. The disparities between the decreases at the Training School and increases in the community are a result of placement outside of the Division's service system, most notably more than 100 deaths and 50 nursing home placements.

Comparatively, the 486 people with developmental disabilities served by the community service providers in 1988 had an average ICAP service score of 74 with a *SD* of 15. In 2004 for 1,752 people the average score decreased to 52. The broad independence scores changed less dramatically. The 1988 average was 495 and the average in 2004 decreased to 440. The average age of individuals served in the community was 35 years in 1988 and 42 years in 2004. More significant was 36 year increase in the age range. In 1988 the ages ranged from 16 to 70, by 2004 the ages of those served ranged from one year to 91 years old. This reflected the movement of older individuals to the community and the implementation of a home and community-based waiver for children.

The average maladaptive score was virtually unchanged but the range increased from 1988 to 2004. The average maladaptive score of people in the community was -9 in 1988, -8 in 2004. The lowest score decreased from -46 in 1988 to -51 in 2004. These results suggest that community programs are serving individuals with broader range of maladaptive scores, but that many are in the normal range.

Table 2
ICAP Demographics In The Institution and Community In 1988 and 2004

	Institution		Community	
	1988	2004	1988	2004
N =	389	93	486	766
Sex				
Male	199	49	298	430
Female	190	44	188	336
Age				
0-17	46	0	5	70
18-21	27	1	50	78
22-39	137	20	296	364
40-61	112	52	124	213
62 or older	67	20	11	41
Mobility				
Walks	269	49	467	658
Non-Ambulatory	120	44	19	94
Family Contact in Month				
Yes	125	16	420	656
No	264	77	66	110
Mental Retardation				
Not Retardation	19	0	107	83
Mild	44	3	218	315
Moderate	45	5	114	171
Severe	47	9	21	81
Profound	233	76	4	77
Not Specified	1	0	22	39

The information in Table 2 shows that between 1988 and 2004 most of the people left the state's only institution. The number of people served in the community tripled as a result of both out-placement from the Training School and the expansion of community services. The Training School served about an equal number of both sexes but the men served in the community made up 61% in 1988 and decreased to 53% in 2004. All but one of the individuals younger than 21 and all but 20 older than 62 years of age left the institution. The community population increased in all age groups but especially in younger and older ages. The institution served some people (36%) who could not walk in 1988 and this reached 53% by 2004. While most of the persons served in the community are mobile, the percentage of people who were non-ambulatory in the community increased from 4% to 17%. In general, the system served people with mental retardation. This became more pronounced by 2004 when everyone in the institution and 1,545 people (88%) in the community did have mental retardation. The remainder had a related condition. The Training School now almost exclusively serves persons with mental retardation. What the table does not show is the widening mix of primary diagnoses being served in 2004, including persons with sensory impairments, autism, and mental illness. There was also an increased need for health related services.

Table 3
Seizures, Required Nurse and/or Physician and Prescribed Medication in the Community and Institution in 1988 and 2004

	1988		2004	
	Inst.	Comm.	Inst.	Comm.
N =	389	486	93	1,752
Seizures				
None or Controlled	274	441	48	1,485
Less than Monthly	43	25	9	91
Monthly	36	1	18	66
Weekly or More Often	36	9	18	110
Not Specified	0	1	0	0
Required nurse/Physician				
Less than Monthly	233	443	36	1,454
Monthly	98	34	42	211
Weekly	36	4	8	64
Daily	12	3	3	13
24 Hour Immediate Access	7	0	3	1
Not Specified	3	2	0	0
Prescribed Medication				
None	66	191	1	392
For Health	115	134	57	467
For Mood, Sleep, Behavior	70	89	34	715
For Epilepsy	131	76	50	451
For Another Reason	166	60	62	682
Not Specified	2	8	0	4

Most of the people served have controlled seizures or none at all, whether they live at the institution and or in the community, but there has been an increase in the percentage of persons in the community who have seizures at least monthly, from 2% (n=10) in 1988 to 23% (n=176) in 2004. By 2004, only 15 people in the institution required weekly or more often than weekly nursing or physician care while the community has 102 people with such medical care needs. All but one person (99%) served in the institution take prescribed medication by 2004 as do 78% of the people served who live in the community. In 2004, health, epilepsy, and other medications lead the list for 56 (60%) of the people who lived in the institution and also were most common with community dwellers. About of 37% of the people served in the institution and 41% of the people served in the community in 2004 took medications for mood, sleep or behavior. This represents little change for the Training School but a substantial increase in the number of persons requiring medications in community programs from 1988. In 1988, about 18% (89 of 486) required these medications compared to 41% (715 of 1752) in 2004.

Table 4
Adaptive Behavior and Problem Behavior in the Community and Institution in 1988 and 2004

	1988		2004	
	Inst.	Comm.	Inst.	Comm.
Adaptive Behavior (fairly or very well)				
Imitates Actions	236	482	29	1,477
Says 10 Words	168	467	27	1,372
Independent Toileting	204	472	15	1,109
Stays in Unfenced Yard	228	479	25	1,098
Speaks in 3-4 Word Sentence	140	449	16	1,120
Dresses Self Completely	161	465	15	171
Crosses Streets Alone	122	383	4	179
Purchase/Count $5 Change	22	209	1	180
Writes Notes or Letters	22	215	0	280
Budgets Money for Week	39	175	0	48
Plans & Prepares Meals	9	90	0	54
Problem Behavior (moderately serious plus)				
Hurts Self	108	47	17	214
Hurts Others	111	46	27	332
Damages Property	161	39	3	117
Disruptive	161	116	16	450
Unusual Repetitive Habits	123	94	9	214
Socially Offensive	16a1	124	6	435
Withdrawn or Inattentive	163	133	1	191
Uncooperative	170	132	17	522

Table 4 displays the adaptive and maladaptive or problem behaviors recorded by the ICAP for the people served in the institution and community for 1988 and 2004. In 2004, the adaptive behavior inventory of the 93 people served in the institution suggests these people needed increased amounts of personal care, adaptive equipment, training, medical care and supervision while some of the community individuals exhibited a wider range of moderate to serious problem behaviors. For example, in 1988, 204 of the 389 (52%) of those at the Training School could independently toilet, but in 2004 the same could be said of only 15 of 93 (16%). The reverse is true for community programs in which 472 of 486 (97%) were independent in 1988, only 63% were in 2004. Similarly, in 1988, 465 of 486 (96%) were independent in dressing; 171 of 1,752 (10%) were independent in

2004. Other adaptive behavior skills, specifically crossing a street alone, counting change, writing notes, budgeting money for the week, and preparing meals, were less prevalent in both groups in 2004 than in 1998. None of those at the Training School in 2004 could demonstrate all these behaviors. In fact, only one could count change and four were capable of crossing a street alone. Among those served in the community, there also was a decline in the absolute number of persons demonstrating these skills, made more remarkable by the fivefold increase in the total number of persons served.

Maladaptive or problem behaviors in the community increased from 40 people to 216 in categories like hurts oneself, hurts others, or damages property. There were 379 people in the community who were rated as having behaviors that were disruptive, or socially offensive, or withdrawn or inattentive, or uncooperative, or having unusual or repetitive habits. About half of the adults who lived in the community in 2004 had one or more moderately serious problem behaviors compared to less than 25% for those behaviors in 1988. The characteristics of those served in the community settings changed between 1988 and 2004, but so have the settings.

Table 5

Challenges and Changes In the Community and Institution in 1988 and 2004

	1988		2004	
	Inst.	Comm.	Inst.	Comm.
Number of Services Available	25	2	30	31
Person Served Annual Cost	$37,782	$8,284	$185,372	$42,789
Ranking of State Per $1,000 Personal Income By DD Funding	4th	23rd	19th	10th
Institutional Per Diem Rate	46th		24th	
Number of People Who Own Their Own Home		0		130
Average Number of People Who Live Together	30	7	5	2
Range of Number of People Who Live Together	10-30	1-15	5-9	1-8
Qualified Mental Retardation Professionals	0	0	11	160
Case Managers – People Served Ratios	35:1	14:1	14:1	16:1

In 1988 there were two community services funded by the state: sheltered workshop and group homes. Across the state, there were 49 community living sites, 28 group homes and 21 apartments. There was an average of seven clients who live at each community site. In 2004, these have expanded to 374 residential settings including 62 adult host families, 191 individuals living in supported apartments, 130 of whom are adults who lease or own their own homes. The most common residential setting is the group home with an average of 4.7 persons per home, but no home with more than 8 persons. Group homes account for 571 adults. Across all community residential settings in 2004, there was an average density of two persons per living site. By way of comparison, the 2000 United States census showed the average household in Wyoming had 2.48 people.

The 2004 Wyoming service array grew into an array of 31 different, supported services replacing the dichotomous vocational and residential funding. In 1988 Wyoming identified no Qualified Mental Retardation Professionals (QMRPs) because there were no ICFs/MR in 1988 but there were 160 by 2004. Case managers (who were also QMRPs in 2004) increased from 45 in 1988 to 160 in 2004. The institution had a ratio of people served to QMRPs of at least 14:1 by 2004 and the community ratio was 16:1. Many states had ratios of 50:1 (Richardson, 1993).

The new or reinforced services in institutional and community settings included western flavored hippotherapy, mealtime management, and adaptive equipment repair. New community services such as skilled nursing and in-home support were added in response to the needs of those served. Transportation was built into the funding for all services, however this may be less supported in actual costs than at the beginning of the waivers. The 2004 community day programming included special education school programming for 546 children (34%), supported employment for 153 (10%), competitive work for 81 (5%), work activity center for 156 (10%), sheltered work for 225 (24%), day habilitation for 380 (24%), and older or retired person's programs for 57 (4%) of the people served.

Besides a wide menu of service choices, the essential factor of rural success in service provision and development was the financial support of the new efforts. Between 1988 and the end of 2004, Wyoming government doubled its overall funding for institutional and community settings, an increase from 40 million to 80 million dollars. Twice as many people were served. The match ratio of the waivers and ICF/MR funding allowed more than half of the cost to be federally supported. At the end of December 2004, there were 175 people with developmental disabilities waiting for waiver services, but Wyoming expected to begin serving them in early 2005.

Wyoming's DOORS (Fortune et al., 2005) individual waiver budget system was the mechanism used to allocate funds to those in the community receiving waiver services. By 2004, average cost for an individual in the community was $42,789; the average cost for an individual served by the Training School was $185,372. Braddock, Hemp, Bachelder, and Fujiura (2004) report Wyoming was ranked 23rd in community services and ranked 4th in institutional care in 1988. Wyoming spent $3.74 per $1,000 of statewide personal income. In 2004, Wyoming was ranked 10th in fiscal effort made toward community programs and ranked 19th at the institution by spending $1.01 per $1,000 of statewide personal income (Rizzolo, Hemp, Braddock, & Pomeranz-Essley, 2004). The low population of the state influences the various statistics, for example, the institution's per diem rate was 48th in the country in 1988. (Mangan, Blake, Prouty, & Lakin, 1994).

Discussion

Although the average service level of those served in the system did not change between 1988 and 2004, ICAP demographics indicate that there was a significant shift in the location of the service. Wyoming has assisted individuals with a broad range of disabilities to move into the community, although the Training School continues to serve individuals with extensive service needs. The people who moved to community settings have been there for an average of twelve years, although the placement record is not perfect. About one percent of the people who left the Training School since the lawsuit was finalized returned for brief periods. This was usually for medical support before returning to the community.

The introduction of the Home and Community Based Waivers brought about significant changes in Wyoming's system of services for persons with developmental disabilities. The relationship of the network of service providers with the people served and their families and with the Division was largely cooperative and personal, although it remains a different service system after than before the waivers. The system of regional service providers who, as a condition of receiving a State contract, were required to serve all persons within their catchment area effectively ended with the waivers. These regional providers, each presently serving more people than the Training School, dominate the system and are in competition with each other in a way never anticipated when the regional system was established in 1979.

Considerable changes have occurred between 1988 and 2004. The number of service providers has dramatically increased, as has the number of persons served in community settings and the costs of supporting them. None of this matters much if no one is satisfied. In 2001, the National Core Indicators Project sampled and interviewed 400 families of the adults with developmental disabilities served across Wyoming, reporting that 93.2% of their family members were happy, which is one important indicator and perhaps the most important indicator. Jobs, smaller residential settings, and increased home ownership are important as well. Can we declare victory? Clearly not. Expectation of what constitutes appropriate services is a moving target, as it should be. Deinstitutionalization was a response to the limitations of institutional services as much as institutionalization was a response to the high expectations for cure that would be the result of concentrated professional intervention. The work is not finished.

This record describes essential aspects of community service use, the characteristics of the people served and their behavioral adjustment for a rural statewide group of people with developmental disabilities. This effort uses the ICAP for group summary information that has descriptive value for telling the story of changing services and persons served in small towns and rural areas. Even basic descriptions in the literature about the people served and service changes in rural states are quite rare. The long-term results of a change in treatment settings and services for a number of people, in this case a switch to community-based services, fit the ICAP's ability to provide measurements across a wide variety of characteristics, skills and service placements, and across a wide range of ages. This effort also provides a confirmation that individuals with a wide range of needs can move from residential institutional care to services in rural communities if there is a wide choice of needed and adequately funded services. The contrasting profile of one state's persons served in the institution and community using the ICAP provides an indication not only of the behavioral functioning of individuals served and relationship to cost but also a description of the attributes the people have and a census of their chosen support services.

References

Bassuk, E. L. & Gerson, S. (1978). Deinstitutionalization and mental health services. *Scientific American, 238,* 46-53.

Bitner, A. (2004). *Wyoming 2004 – Just the Facts!* Cheyenne, WY: Wyoming Department of Administration and Information, Economic Analysis Division. http://eadiv.state.wy.u

Braddock, D., Hemp, R., Bachelder, L., & Fujiura, G. (1993). *National retardation/developmental disability expenditure data base.* Chicago: University of Illinois at the Chicago University Affiliated Program.

Brown, M. C. et al. (1986). *The developmental disabilities profile: Final report on the design, development & testing of the core instrument.* Albany: New York State Office of Mental Retardation and Developmental Disabilities.

Bruininks, R. H., Hill, B. K., Weatherman, R. F., & Woodcock, R. W. (1986). *Inventory for client and agency planning.* Chicago, IL: Riverside Publishing Company.

Campbell, E. M., Fortune, J., Frisch, J. K., Heal, L. W., Heinlein, K. B., Lynch R. M., et al. (2005). Predictors of expenditures in western states. In J. R. Stancliffe & K. C. Lakin (Eds.), *Costs and outcomes community services for people with intellectual disabilities* (pp.175-201). Baltimore: Paul H. Brookes.

Chapin, R. (1991, June). *Targeted reimbursement for long term care services for persons with developmental disabilities.* Proceedings of a forum sponsored by the Office of Social Policy Analysis, School of Social Work, (pp. 1-102). Lawrence, KS: The University of Kansas.

Chen, T., Bruininks, R. H., Lakin, C. L., & Hayden, M. (1993). Personal competencies and community participation in small community residential programs: a multiple discriminant analysis. *American Journal on Mental Retardation, 98,* 390-399.

DeStefano, L. (1992). Inventory for client and agency planning. In D. J. Keyser & R. C. Sweetland (Eds), *Test Critiques, 9,* (pp. 319-331). Austin, TX: Pro-ed.

Emerson, E. (2004). Deinstitutionalization in England. *Journal of Intellectual & Developmental Disability, 29,* 79-84.

Fortune, J., Heinlein, K. B., & Fortune, B. (1995). Changing the shape of the service population. *European Journal of Mental Disability,* 2(8), 20-37.

Fortune, J., Smith, G., Campbell, E. M., Clabby, R. T., Heinlein, K. H., Lynch, R. M., et al. (2005). Individual budgets according to individual needs: The Wyoming DOORS system. In J. R. Stancliffe & K. C. Lakin (Eds.), *Costs and outcomes of community services for people with intellectual disabilities* (pp. 241-262). Baltimore: Paul H. Brookes.

Haugen, J. (1990, June). *Identifying residential and day programs for adults with developmental disabilities: An application of discriminant analysis.* Paper presented at the Annual Meeting of the American Association on Mental Retardation, Atlanta, GA.

Jacobson, J. W., Sersen, E., & Schwartz, A. A. (1984). Characteristics and adaptive behaviors of New York's group home occupants. *Perspectives and progress in mental retardation, 1,* 373-382.

Jahoda, A. & Markova, I. (2004). Coping with social stigma: People with intellectual disabilities moving from institutions and family home. *Journal of Intellectual Disability Research, 48,* 719-729.

Johnson, R. (1989). Review of the inventory for client and agency planning. In J. C. Conoley & J. J. Kramer (Eds.), *Tenth Mental Measurements Yearbook* (pp. 384-385). Lincoln: University of Nebraska Press.

Kim, S., Larson, S. A. & Lakin, K. C. (2001). Behavioral outcomes of deinstitutionalization for people with intellectual disabilities: A review of studies conducted between 1980 and 1999. *Journal of Intellectual & Developmental Disability, 26,* 35-50.

Lakin, K. C. (2004). Residential services for persons with developmental disabilities: Status and trends through 2003. Minneapolis: University of Minnesota, Center for Residential Services and Community Living Institute on Community Integration/UAP.

Lakin, K. C., Blake, E. M., Prouty, R. W., Mangan, T., & Bruininks, R. H. (1993). *Residential services for persons with developmental disabilities: Status and trends through 1991.* Minneapolis: University of Minnesota, Center for Residential Services and Community Living Institute on Community Integration/UAP.

Lakin, K. C., Bruininks, R. H. & Sigford, B. B. (1981). Introduction. In R. H. Bruininks, C. E. Meyers, B. B. Sigford, & K. C. Lakin (Eds), *Deinstitutionalization and community adjustment of mentally retarded people* (AAMD Monograph, No. 4). Washington, DC: American Association on Mental Deficiency.

Lakin, K. C., Prouty, B., Blake, E., and Mangan, T. (1993). Persons with mental retardation and related conditions in state institutions: Tends and projections. *Policy Research Briefs, 5(1).*

Leal, L. (1992). Inventory for client and agency planning. In D. J. Keyser & R. C. Sweetland (Eds), *Test Critiques, 8,* (pp. 290-299). Austin, TX: Pro-ed.

Mangan, T., Blake, E. M., Prouty, R. W., & Lakin, L. C. (1994). *Residential services for persons with mental retardation and related conditions: status and trends through 1993.* Minneapolis: University of Minnesota, Research and Training Center on Residential Services and Community Living Institute on Community Integration (UAP).

McGrew, K. S., Ittenbach, R. F. Bruininks, R. H., & Hill, B. K. (1991). Factor structure of maladaptive behavior across the lifespan of persons with mental retardation. *Research in Developmental Disabilities, 12,* 181-199.

McGrew, K. S., Bruininks, R. H. & Thurlow, M. L. (1992). Relationships between measures of adaptive functioning and community adjustment for adults with mental retardation. *Exceptional Children, 58,* 517-529.

Palmer, R. (1974). *Prediction of work performance and work adjustment in mentally retarded adults.* Uppsala, Sweden: Scandinavian University Books.

Perry, J. & Felce, D. (2003). Quality of life outcomes for people with intellectual disabilities living in staffed community housing services: a stratified random sample of statutory, voluntary and private agency provision. *Journal of Applied Research in Intellectual Disability, 16,* 11-28.

Quinsey, V. L., Book, A., & Skilling, T. A. (2004). A follow-up of deinstitutionalized men with intellectual disabilities and histories of antisocial behaviour. *Journal of Applied Research in Intellectual Disabilities, 17,* 243-253.

Richardson, S. K. (1993, November). *Approaches to quality under home and community-based services waivers* (pp. 60-61). Washington, DC: Health Care Financing Administration, Medicaid Bureau.

Spreat, S., & Conrad, J. W. (2002). The impact on deinstitutionalization on family contact. *Research in Developmental Disabilities, 23,* 202-211.

Thompson, J. R., & et al. (2004). *Supports Intensity Scale.* Washington, DC: American Association of Mental Retardation.

Walker, R. A., & Prazak G. (1989, April). *Program evaluation for residential services programs.* Tucson, AZ: Commission on Accreditation of Rehabilitation Facilities.

Wikoff, R. L. (1989). Review of the inventory for client and agency planning. In J. C. Conoley & J. J. Kramer (Eds.), *Tenth Mental Measurements Yearbook* (pp. 385-387). Lincoln, NE: University of Nebraska Press.

Wolfensberger, W. (1972). *Principle of normalization in human services.* Toronto, Canada: National Institute on Mental Retardation.

World Almanac (2005). *World Almanac and Book of Facts.* New York: Author.

Young, L., & Ashman, A. F. (2004). Deinstitutionalization for older adults with severe mental retardation: Results from Australia. *American Journal of Mental Retardation, 109,* 397-412.

Young, L., Ashman, A., Sigafoos, J., & Grevell, P. (2001). Closure of the Challinor Centre II: An extended report on 95 individuals after 12 months of community living. *Journal of Intellectual & Developmental Disabilities, 26,* 51-66.

Community Support Teams: A Collaborative Home-Based Support Model

Rebecca L. Mandal, Ph.D.; Jim LeVelle, Ph.D.; Diane Wilson, LCSW; and Susan Orman, M.S.H.C.M., M.S.N., R.N.; Judith Hill-Weld, M.S.; James LeVelle, Ph.D.; Diane Wilson, L.C.S.W.

In late 2002, Louisiana's state Office for Citizens with Developmental Disabilities developed Community Support Teams (CSTs) to address the needs of children and adults in the community who have co-occurring developmental disabilities and psychiatric disorders. This event was spurred by an increase in the number of referrals to developmental centers involving people with mental health needs. At the time, it became clear that many of the people referred could succeed in the community with access to more intensive behavioral and/or psychiatric supports. However, to achieve this goal a new system of supports had to be developed.

Several obstacles made this task especially difficult. While Louisiana is a culturally rich state, it continues to be economically poor. Louisiana ranks 47th in the nation in average personal income and 4th in the number of people living at poverty level (Statistical Abstracts of the United States, 2004). This, in turn, translates to a meager state budget and customers who are less likely to have the income, insurance, or transportation necessary to access supports. Second, because Louisiana is primarily a rural state, it becomes challenging to develop accessible supports. Of the four and a half million people living in the state, approximately two-thirds live in the southern regions of the state. There are many large geographical areas where psychiatric and psychological services are not easily accessed, especially in the northern part of the state. Many people would need to travel several hours to reach supports. In summary, new supports for people with co-occurring conditions would have to be developed on a limited budget yet provide intensive supports, even in very remote areas of the state.

Initially, Louisiana considered developing Assertive Community Treatment teams (ACT) (Allness & Knoedler, 2003), but this option exceeded the current budget and relied on a medical model. As an alternative the current community support model was developed. This model relies on Community Support Teams (CSTs) to provide intensive quality supports for people with co-occurring conditions who are at risk of losing their desired community living option because of their behavior. It does not provide the 24 hour crisis intervention an ACT team usually provides, although crisis plans are developed using available resources, and phone assistance is available 24 hours a day. Currently, Louisiana has nine teams serving all regions of the state.

Community Support Model

The community support model relies on CSTs to develop positive behavior supports using an approach that is person-centered, collaborative, and evidence-based. A multimodal transdisciplinary team approach is used to understand the person's needs from multiple perspectives including: behavior analytical, a biopsychosocial, and a neuropsychiatric viewpoint (Griffiths, Gardner, & Nugent, 1999). CSTs provide supports that may include brief consultation, assessment, behavior support planning, psychiatric services, family support and education, coordination of health services, and other supports, as needed, to support a person's ability to live successfully in the community.

CST services are provided in community settings in which people live, such as in their home, work place, school, or other locations. This is beneficial for many reasons: transportation concerns are resolved, appointments are seldom missed, natural environments can be assessed, the family's culture and values can be better understood (Koegel, Koegel, & Dunlap, 1996; Lucyshyn, Dunlap, & Albin, 2002), and functional skills can be taught in the natural settings for better generalization (Stokes & Baer, 1977). This also allows for increased opportunities to collaborate with various stakeholders who are involved in the life of the person receiving supports.

When developing strategies with people and their families and/or direct support workers, there can be considerable variance in the assessments and supports that they may choose. While people are encouraged to participate fully, some people do not want to participate in comprehensive assessments and intensive interventions. However, these people can often gain benefits through a consultative approach.

Team Composition

The CSTs consist of a licensed doctoral psychologist, a psychological associate or assistant, a board certified psychiatrist, a licensed clinical social worker, and a registered nurse. All positions are full-time, except that some teams have a registered nurse for 20 hours a week. In addition, psychiatrists only provide services 4-8 hours per week. Psychiatrists also vary in the services that they provide, as some psychiatrists act as consultants while others prescribe medication. When a psychiatrist does not prescribe, collaborative relationships are built between public mental health agencies and private psychiatrists. This can sometimes be beneficial because the dialogue helps to educate professionals in the community about developmental disabilities and thus builds service capacity for this underserved population.

When recruiting team members, efforts have been made to acquire qualified staff with experience in serving people with developmental disabilities. This has sometimes been difficult in rural areas. For example, a strong background in behavioral analysis has been sought for psychologist positions, but this has not always been possible. Ongoing training in behavioral analysis, ethics, and other topics are provided on an ongoing basis for all team members, thus allowing each to continue learning about the other disciplines on the team. The state also supports the CSTs in obtaining continuing education units for their individual professions.

Although the CSTs provide services in community settings (e.g., home, work, school), most are operated from the regional offices that are responsible for serving people with developmental disabilities in their geographical areas. These locations have been invaluable because staff within the regional offices are often knowledgeable about the people and resources in their area.

Criteria for CST Services

The following outlines the criteria for people seeking CST services. All the criteria must be met in order to participate in the program.

1. A statement from Louisiana's Office for Citizens with Developmental Disabilities indicating that the person is eligible for state supports and services for people with developmental disabilities.
2. A pattern of severe and recurrent challenging behaviors that can be characterized by one or more of the following statements:
   a. The person's behavior is potentially harmful to oneself or others (e.g., self-injurious behavior, physical aggression).
   b. The person's behavior significantly impinges upon the rights of others (e.g., property destruction, theft, etc.)
3. No other professional resources are available to address the person's psychiatric or behavioral needs. (Note: This excludes people living in ICF/MR homes or institutions, or other facilities where agencies are responsible for meeting the behavioral needs of the people they serve).
4. The person is at-risk of losing his or her current community placement because of their behavior.

The CSTs are not designed to be a crisis intervention service. Therefore, if any of the following are present the CST will seek additional supports with the help of the regional office.

- suicidal or homicidal behavior
- health status significantly reduced, requiring long-term care
- other life-threatening behaviors (e.g., extreme physical aggression likely to lead to serious harm, repetitive fire setting, planned or group violence)
- forcible and violent sexual acts
- clear and persistent inability, given developmental abilities, to maintain physical safety and/or access safety resources within his or her environment
- behavior which is likely to lead to serious or extreme risk of victimization, abuse, or neglect
- high intensity support level score (>3) on the Child and Adolescent Level of Care Utilization System (CALOCUS). The CALOCUS is a risk assessment tool utilized to determine the level of crisis for an individual which is conducted on-site at the initial intake meeting (Klaehn, O'Malley, Vaughan, Sowers, & Kroeger, 2002).

CST Support Capacity

The CSTs serve people of all ages and in all parts of the state. The state is divided into nine Medicaid regions, and there is one CST per region. Most of the regions can take up to 2 hours to drive across and each CST is expected to support 10-30 people, depending upon the intensity of the needs of the persons served and the number of active CST members available. For example, if consultation is desired by a majority of the people receiving CST's services, then the CST can serve more people. In comparison, if the CST is serving people with very intensive service needs, then few people can be served by the CST. To this date, no team has actively served more than 26 people at any given time, and the average number receiving intensive supports by each CST is approximately twelve per month. The average number of brief consultations provided by each team is approximately 16 per month. Brief consultations involve short-term services (i.e., 1-4 sessions) that characteristically do not require all the disciplines on the team.

Working with People, Families, and Providers

An important component of the community support model is the use of positive behavior supports for assisting a person to reach their desired goals. This approach focuses on enhancing the person's quality of life in all areas, (i.e., home, school, work, and other community settings) while building on strengths and decreasing challenging behaviors (Carr et al., 2002). The CSTs collaborate with the person, their family, professionals, and others in the person's circle of support to create a person-centered plan that includes behavioral and psychiatric supports. It is the CST's responsibility to explain the benefits of assessment and therapeutic options in a manner that helps a person understand the time commitment, efforts, difficulties, and expectancies of the therapeutic process. CST services may vary in intensity based on the willingness of a person to participate. For example, some family members are reluctant to have therapists in their homes or may believe that data collection is too laborious or unnecessary. People are not dropped from services for these reasons. The CST works with the family to obtain as much progress as possible.

All participants receive a Personal Outcomes Assessment (POA, The Council on Quality and Leadership in Supports for People with Disabilities, 2000) to help the team identify and obtain an understanding of the individual's desires and goals in life. This information is considered essential to treatment planning because it allows everyone in the person's circle of support to have an understanding of what the person's goals are while designing ways to make the goals achievable.

For most participants, a functional behavioral assessment is conducted to identify the function of challenging behaviors. Target behaviors are selected based on how much they interfere with a person's ability to reach their own desired outcomes, as obtained from the POA. The functional behavioral assessment includes the identification of the person's strengths, preferred activities, antecedents, setting events, consequences, and other factors. The goal of this approach is to identify the function of the challenging behavior, then reduce the behavior by creating a positive, proactive environment and teaching replacement skills for the challenging behavior using evidence based interventions (Carr et al., 2002). In addition, a psychosocial assessment, health care screening, and psychiatric review, if necessary, are conducted to complete the bio-psychosocial assessment. These assessments are then carefully linked to supports and treatment planning with the goal of improving the person's quality of life (Carr et al., 2002; Lucyshyn et al., 2002).

Supporting People in Rural and Urban Areas

Person-centered planning and positive behavioral supports are important, but effective community supports also rely on competent professionals with expertise in serving people with developmental disabilities. This can often be problematic in urban areas, but is even more difficult in rural areas. As stated above, Louisiana is a largely rural state and psychiatric or behavioral services may be several hours away for many people. Others lack transportation to get there or the person with a developmental disability does not travel well. This is remedied by having the CSTs travel to the person's home, work, school, and other places in the community where they live. This approach is essential for three primary reasons. First, if supports are not brought to the person it is probable that they will not receive services and will not be able to remain in their current residence. Second, providing services where the challenging problem exists helps the CSTs observe and understand the context of both positive and self-defeating behaviors for the individual and the family. Third, assessment and treatment in natural settings can lead to improved generalization (Stokes & Baer, 1972).

Inter-agency Collaboration

One important function of the CSTs is to collaborate with and coordinate services provided through various agencies. For example, many of the individuals served are school-age, thus it becomes necessary to work with the local school districts to support these children. Although school districts may employ school psychologists, behavior analysts, and behavior shaping specialists to provide behavioral services to children in their school district, ideally the children will receive continuity of services across home and school settings. The CSTs work to bridge the gap between home and school with the goal of an effective treatment plan which can be put into action in both settings. Both parties can communicate and work together in the best interest of the student and increase the likelihood the child will succeed at both home and school.

In addition to schools, multiple agencies often provide services to the person. The CSTs coordinate the efforts of various stakeholders so that everyone is working together. This requires skills in collaborating with and educating the community so that there is increased awareness about the needs of people with developmental disabilities. Ideally, this will lead to greater capacity in the community while providing an improved system of supports for the person relying on the CSTs.

One example of a CST developing inter-agency collaboration involved a ten year old boy we will call Steve and his foster family. Steve was referred to the CST because of his physical aggression and "violent homicidal and suicidal behaviors" and was at-risk of losing his current placement with his fifth foster family. The school he was attending was unable to manage his behavior without the presence of several male staff who were prepared to restrain him if an episode should occur. It was soon learned that Steve was served by 12 different agencies and that these agencies were not communicating with one another.

A meeting involving all 12 agencies was soon held and it was revealed that Steve had been admitted to an in-patient psychiatric hospital for four months without his school being notified. At the end of his stay, he was brought back to school to begin class, yet there had been no communication of this plan between his foster parent and the school district. Other agencies were equally in the dark about facets of Steve's care although it often affected their ability to serve him. By the end of the meeting, many complaints had been vented but little had been done to support Steve.

Oddly, when the CST met with Steve they found a boy who was not as difficult or as dangerous as had been described. The primary problem was that he was not receiving consistent supports across systems. To begin the process of coordinating a consistent system of support, the CST established communication between the school, the local mental health center, the foster parent, and other agencies. Communication and collaboration between all parties was greatly increased, the continuity of his supports across the systems was enhanced, and Steve's behavior rapidly improved and stabilized. By the next inter-agency meeting, discussion revolved around Steve's needs, instead of complaints about past misunderstandings. Four months later Steve was doing well, and his foster family was happy for him to stay with them indefinitely.

In contrast to working with multiple agencies, the CSTs sometime cannot locate agencies to provide needed supports that may enhance a person's quality of life, especially in rural areas. Thus, the CSTs investigate supports and services that can be brought into the home, school, or work setting. For example, one CST was working with an adult individual who was deaf and who had minimal sign language skills. In order to communicate his needs more effectively, he, his family, and his staff needed to learn more sign language. The CST found a resource that provided sign language on the computer using an actual person demonstrating the words and phrases being taught. This resource was given to the family and staff for their utilization and as a result, the individual's ability as well as his staff's ability improved.

In other situations, the CSTs have communicated with regional offices and providers to extend supports by other agencies to serve people with developmental disabilities. The CSTs offer to assist these agencies in learning about developmental disabilities and provide training to the agency staff. For example, one CST attended a community provider fair and began talking to a private agency that provided speech, occupational, and physical therapy. This agency accepted Medicaid/Medicare and had traditionally not provided services to people with developmental disabilities.

After discussing the lack of services in the region for people with developmental disabilities, this agency indicated that with training they would agree to serve people with developmental disabilities in this region. On other occasions where private services can not be located in the area, the CSTs request professional services from the developmental centers to serve people in their community.

Support Teams

The CSTs work to be valuable members of a person's Support Team and if the person does not have a Support Team, the CST will create one. The Support Teams include the CST, the person receiving services, family members, advocates, direct support providers, and support coordinators, and anyone else that the person chooses to invite. The Support Team reviews Personal Outcome Assessments and professional evaluations to identify the person's needs, strengths, and preferences to develop a Plan of Support. This plan encompasses all aspects of the person's life. Within this plan, the CST includes strategies that the Support Team agrees to carry out. The CST also develops a Team Support Plan that outlines for all team members the plan for providing supports for a person. The Team Support Plan provides a detailed description of the supports and treatment strategies that will be implemented. This plan includes the following:

- **Interim strategies**: These are strategies that are often implemented during an assessment phase to prevent a situation from quickly becoming a crisis.
- **Identified Needs:** These needs are based on the evaluative information and Support Team discussions.
- **Long and short term goals/objectives:** The goals and objectives are specific and measurable functional outcomes to be achieved through the selected supports and treatments.
- **Supports/treatments**: Specific supports or treatment interventions that will be employed.
- **Responsibilities:** The plan identifies who will take responsibility for different facets of the plan including provision of supports and the implementation of strategies.
- **Training and treatment integrity measures:** The plan outlines the competency-based training and treatment integrity measures that will be provided throughout treatment.
- **Success criteria and criteria for discontinuation of CST supports and services:** Since goals and objectives are identified and established in the beginning of the plan, success criteria are based on these goals. Discontinuation of CST supports is clearly stated in the plan so that all are aware of the expectations of the plan from the beginning of treatment.
- **Crisis strategies:** This includes clear strategies for avoiding crises and for responding to crises in order to minimize risks to the person and those around them.

The person receiving supports and those supporting him or her, generally receive a succinct plan stemming from the Team Support Plan that clearly describes the strategies that they will be responsible for implementing.

Education and Successful Outcomes

In order to produce successful outcomes in a person's natural environment it becomes paramount that collaborative partnerships are developed when planning and implementing strategies. After all, it is the person and the person's circle of support that will provide most of the supports and strategies that are developed, and they are the ones that will maintain positive outcomes long after the CSTs have gone. For this reason, educating the person and those who support them is an important part of providing effective supports.

Education can also be more difficult than it sounds, and developing effective strategies for teaching information and skills can be complex. The therapist must recognize the large number of variables that can affect learning activities such as the rate of learning and retention of those being taught, cultural expectations (Albin, Lucyshyn, Horner, & Flannery, 1996), level of education, myths about behavior, resistance to change, motivation, and so on. Therefore, the CSTs are encouraged to be innovative, to consider multiple methods for teaching and maintaining skills, and to use competency-based measures (Reid & Parsons, 2002).

Methods for teaching family, staff, and others how to implement strategies usually include didactic presentation and role-play (Reid & Parson, 2002). However, PowerPoint presentations with handouts, pre- and post- tests to determine retention of information, feedback during integrity checks, book recommendations, conference notifications, resource references, and other tools may be used to help people truly understand how strategies are supposed to work and to learn more about a person's disability. Repeated training and feedback must be provided frequently, so that people do not lose their skills. The frequency of this training varies, depending on the abilities of those who are implementing the strategies.

Many of the educational activities provided by the CSTs focus on teaching the skills that will impact the rate or intensity of a person's challenging behaviors. An emphasis on teaching positive skills is a primary component of providing positive behavior supports and is generally essential to achieving long term gains (Carr et al., 2002). The CSTs include educational objectives for teaching replacement behaviors that are functionally equivalent to challenging behaviors. However, the CSTs take a broader perspective and will often include additional skills training activities that are not directly related to the person's challenging behavior, but rather are important to the person's overall quality of life. In some instances, this has been surprisingly relevant to the occurrence of challenging behaviors.

For example, Lenny was referred to the CST because his aggressive behavior and "unwillingness" to care for his health were jeopardizing his ability to continue living in his own apartment. Lenny was a young man in his 20's with mild intellectual disabilities who had many skills for living well in his own apartment. He was also irritable much of the time and had a love of food that led to morbid obesity and hypertension. His overeating appeared to be detrimental to his quality of life.

The CST assessed Lenny's preferences, his understanding of nutrition, and the contents of his refrigerator and pantry. They found that Lenny had little understanding of nutrition and the causes and dangers of obesity and hypertension. The CST taught both Lenny and his staff the importance of a healthy diet using the Food Guide Pyramid and taught some simple methods for determining appropriate portions of food. He was also given a cookbook with recipes low in fat and sodium, and, with his input, a shopping list was developed. The importance of exercise was also taught, and times for daily walks were scheduled. Staff were also taught the importance of reinforcing Lenny's "good decisions."

Follow-up to the training involved re-educating Lenny and his staff when poor food choices were made. Hypertension, blood pressure, and medications were monitored by his physician. Lenny began to understand the importance of healthy eating and soon embraced his new lifestyle. He purchased healthy meals and bought a special grill that decreased the amount of fat in the meats he liked. He also began substituting low fat snacks for the cupcakes that he "loved." As a result, Lenny's health and disposition improved, and he continues to live in his own apartment.

Problems Encountered and Resolutions

Lack of Resources

People in rural areas often lack the supports they need. This diminishes the person's quality of life and often leads to challenging behaviors. People who live with pain or illness without treatment, live in isolation without access to rewarding activities, or lack assistance to meet their daily needs can often show signs of depression or anxiety and behaviors such as aggression, self-injury, or property destruction are not uncommon (Bailey & Pyles, 1989).

The CSTs have taken on the responsibility for the searching for supports when important services are missing. This can often involve calling many providers until the needed supports could be located or recruited to the area. Other times supports were located through the Internet, hospitals, and other state agencies. The CSTs also utilize Louisiana's five Resource Centers, which are located throughout the state, with each focusing on different specialty areas or professions. The five specialty Resource Centers are: Aging; Community Inclusion; Medical and Dental Supports; Nutritional, Physical and Nursing Supports; and Psychiatric and Behavior Supports. The Resource Centers were designed to utilize existing resources or aid in the development of supports so that individuals with developmental disabilities have an enhanced quality of life. Resource Centers achieve this by identifying the overall needs of the people with developmental disabilities across the state in the specialty areas. The Resource Centers can then increase and enhance the existing supports in the community by utilizing expertise within the service system to educate and build community capacity. In addition to Resource Centers, the CSTs may also seek assistance in the community from area developmental centers, such as nutrition, occupational therapy, and physical therapy consults. These options have been utilized many times and can be very effective.

Resistance to Therapy

The CSTs commonly provide supports that are developed and implemented in collaboration with family members and/or staff. Despite the use of the collaborative approach, the CSTs continue to encounter resistance to the application of behavioral recommendations. Even though families and provider staff initially appear anxious to receive CST services, many appear to have a misunderstanding about how changes can come about and the effort that may be involved for behavioral strategies to be effective. Sometimes it is expected that the CST will come and "do all the work" necessary to "fix the person." To address this issue, the CSTs begin the intake session by explaining the process of assessment, planning, and successful treatment, including the necessity of their role in implementing strategies. It is emphasized that this a learning process for the person receiving supports and everyone else involved. Realistic expectations are also addressed so that people know that challenging behaviors may get worse before they get better (e.g., extinction burst, reactions to new rules, etc.) and that consistency in applying the selected strategies is of major importance. These instructions are repeated as needed and proper implementation of strategies is socially reinforced by the CST, and, hopefully, programmatic success also encourages continued implementation. People are also informed that systematic revisions in strategies may occur as needed if a plan is not working as expected or it becomes logistically unwieldy to implement.

In one situation, one of the CSTs worked with two parents who were resistant to the behavioral strategies planned for their two children with autism. Despite helping to develop the treatment strategies and effectively training direct support staff, the parents did not follow the plan. The importance of consistent implementation was explained, but this continued until the CST tactfully proposed a behavioral contract wherein an agreement was signed to implement the strategies.

Social Isolation

Social isolation is a problem that is especially common in rural areas. It is often difficult for people to find companionship in urban areas, but in rural areas the opportunities are much more limited. People who experience social isolation may not learn social norms or may respond to others in a manner that is not appropriate. This can sometimes be construed as frightening, dangerous, promiscuous, bossy, or laughable. In some situations, this has lead to responses that upset the person and aggressive behaviors follow, producing a cyclical process of problems for the person in the community. When social isolation is noted as a problem area, the CSTs try to carefully explain to the Support Team that the importance of the person being included in community activities is central to the development of social networks and the understanding of social norms. One man, Gabriel, who was served by one CST lived in his own home and had staff to provide supports on a 24 hour basis. He had previously lived in an institutional setting and lacked skills needed for interacting appropriately with others in the community. Staff were instructed to take Gabriel to personally pay his rent, electricity, and water bills to those he owed. He began to have regular interaction with those individuals he encountered. Next, Gabriel began eating at local restaurants and shopping at the grocery store where he talked to people who waited on him in these businesses. Over a period of time Gabriel was greeted by the employees when he entered their places of business. He later became a part of a work crew who went into the community to provide janitorial services, where he interacted with more people in the community. He also ventured out to garage sales and to his neighbors, visiting them from time to time. In this way the community was utilized to provide Gabriel with a much needed and satisfying level of interaction with others.

Outcome Measures

Establishment of the CSTs was largely influenced by the need to reduce referrals and admissions to institutional environments. However, neither referrals nor admissions could be used as a determinant of success for the CSTs' program, because these variables have not been stable in the past, and are influenced by other factors beyond the scope of the program (e.g., court orders, regional resources, and custodial parent's request). A better measure to indicate the success of the program was the percentage of people receiving CST services who were not referred to more restrictive, institutional environments. This seems appropriate, in part, because the people served by the program have the same characteristics as those who are referred directly to the institution, and all were in imminent jeopardy of losing their home placement.

The CSTs have served approximately 305 individuals throughout the state since their inception in July 2003 and extending to February of 2005. When the CSTs report that an individual has been "served" by the team this means that an individual receives services from all disciplines on the team and has a Team Support Plan. In other words, these are not people who are considered under the brief consultation umbrella. Of the 305 individuals served by the CSTs, 85% were not referred for more restrictive placement and are currently living in their communities. We have concluded from the data that the CSTs are effectively providing a necessary service to those individuals, a service that did not exist prior to the creation of the CSTs.

Sixty-two percent of the individuals served by the CSTs are children, whereas approximately 38% are adults. Serving children with disabilities is beneficial for a number of reasons. First, serving children allows the CSTs to help provide interventions earlier, before difficult behavior may become unmanageable and then possibly result in a more intrusive placement. Thus, early prevention is the key.

Secondly, the CSTs are able to build collaborative relationships with school systems so that the child may receive consistent services across home and school settings. Third, the CSTs are able to come into contact with several agencies serving children and are able to help develop and educate these agencies about developmental disabilities, thus building more community awareness about disabilities. Fourth, these collaborative relationships help establish working relationships with other agencies, thus increasing communication. For example, one CST was working with an agency that provides in-patient psychiatric and intensive behavioral supports for adolescents. The CST received a referral from this agency for an adolescent who lived in a rural area where there were not adequate supports available. The adolescent was served for 8 months through the CST and services were successfully discontinued. Later in the year, the CST was serving an adolescent who needed more intensive services than the CST could provide in the community. The in-patient agency worked with the CST on providing intensive services for the adolescent and then ultimately discharged him back to the CST, which continued to provide services for the child in the community. Subsequently, continuity of care was obtained for this individual and benefited him by allowing him to continue to live in the community with the help of the two agencies.

In addition to the individuals that receive services from all the disciplines on the CSTs, the CSTs also routinely perform brief consultations for other agencies or families overseeing the welfare of individuals with developmental disabilities in the community. Since the CSTs are not able (due to an average of three to five staff) to provide full services to many people living in the community, often consults are performed to assist these individuals with issues that arise. For example, one CST was recently consulted about "Rachel" who lost a personal care attendant whom she had been very close to and her mother had been placed in a nursing home. She became very depressed, neglecting her self care and the cleaning of her apartment, putting her at imminent risk of losing her home. She was also jeopardizing her job by verbally lashing out at others. The CST advised staff from her provider agency to obtain more PCA services, obtain grief counseling, and schedule a visit with her current psychiatrist. The provider agency staff complied with recommendations, and the individual was able to resume her ability to function within a few weeks.

Another example of a brief consultation is when the CSTs provide services in the person's home on a short term basis (one to two visits) to provide additional behavioral recommendations as needed. Brief consultations of this type are performed in a variety of situations, and as a result many individuals have been able to avert the loss of their job, home, and personal staff. The CSTs view this as a valuable addition to the services they routinely perform because, due to the short term nature of these services, the CSTs are able to assist a greater number of individuals living in the community setting. The CSTs provide an average of 16 brief consultations each month. If this were calculated over a one year period, it would be concluded that the CSTs are providing abbreviated services to over 190 individuals, in addition to those that receive full CST services.

Other data to examine is the cost savings to the state for the services being provided. It is estimated that the cost of serving one person in a state funded intermediate care facility is approximately $106,000 (Rizzolo, Hemp, Braddock, & Pomeranz-Essley, 2004). Each CST receives an average of $240,000 per year to cover salaries and travel expenses. The statewide CST program costs a total of approximately 2 million dollars a years. If just 20 of the people served per year were diverted from institutional settings by the CSTs, the program will have paid for itself.

Funding is, however, one aspect of the CSTs that needs further investigation. As in most states, the funding that is given to state agencies continues to decrease over time. There is less money for the increasing number of people that need services, and the Louisiana Office for Citizens with Developmental Disabilities is no exception. The instability of being given state general funds is forcing the CSTs to seek sources for other income to support the teams. Medicaid is one option that has surfaced. Approximately 71% of those being served by the CSTs have Medicaid or are Medicaid eligible. The monies generated from Medicaid funding may help off-set some of the cost of CSTs so that less money is needed from the state general funds. Additionally, federal and state grants are another funding option that may help temporarily secure funding for the CSTs.

Another difficulty that is encountered by the current CSTs is that they have reached individual support capacity. Several CSTs have people awaiting their services and given that each person is served by the team for 8-18 months, there is a considerable amount of time before other people can be served. Subsequently, more teams also means more money. Until a viable solution can be found for funding, the people awaiting services from the CSTs will continue to remain stable or increase.

Despite funding and a limited number of teams, the CSTs are providing a much needed service to people with developmental disabilities living in the community, particularly in rural areas where supports did not previously exist. Bringing the services to the community has shown other benefits as well. It offers the therapist the opportunity to observe in natural settings, to better understand the person and his or her family, and to treat challenging behaviors in the natural environment which avoids concerns with generalization. In addition, providing services in the community allows for collaboration between the multiple agencies that serve this population. This increases the likelihood that people will have continuity of care as well as consistency across multiple settings like home, work, or school. In conclusion, CSTs seem to be effectively meeting the needs of children and adults in the community who have co-occurring developmental disabilities and psychiatric disorders.

References

Albin, R. W., Lucyshyn, J. M., Horner, R. H., & Flannery, K. B. (1996). Contextual fit for behavioral support plans: A model for "Goodness of Fit." In L. K. Koegel, R. L. Koegel,

& G. Dunlap (Eds), *Positive behavioral support: Including people with difficult behaviors in the community* (pp 81-98). Baltimore: Brookes.

Allness, D. & Knoedler, W. (2003). *National program standards for ACT teams (2003 revision).* Arlington, VA: NAMI.

Bailey, J.dS., & Pyles, D. A. M. (1989). *Behavioral Diagnostics, Monographs of the American Association on Mental Retardation, 12,* 85-106.

Carr, E. G., Dunlap, G., Horner, R. H., Koegel, R. L., Turnbull, A. P., Sailor, W., et al. (2002). Positive behavior support: Evolution of an applied science. *Journal of Positive Behavior Interventions, 4(1),* 4-16, 20.

Griffiths, D. M., Gardner, W. I., & Nugent, J. A, (1999). *Behavioral support: Individual centered interventions, A multimodal functional approach.* Kingston, NY: NADD Press.

Klaehn, R., O'Malley, K., Vaughan, T., Sowers, W., & Kroeger, K. (2002). *CALOCUS User's Manual.* American Academy of Child and Adolescent Psychiatry.

Koegel, L. K., Koegel, R. L., & Dunlap, G. (Eds.) (1996). *Positive behavioral support: Including people with difficult behavior in the community.* Baltimore, MD: Paul H. Brookes Publishers.

Lucyshyn, J. M., Horner, R. H., Dunlap, G., Albin, R. W., & Ben, K. R. (2002). Positive behavior support with families. In J. M. Lucyshyn, G., Dunlap, & R. W. Albin, (Eds.), *Families and positive behavior support* (pp. 3-43). Baltimore, MD: Paul H. Brookes Publishing Co.

Reid, D. H. & Parsons, M. B. (2002). *Working with staff to overcome challenging behavior among people who have severe disabilities.* Morgantown, NC: Habilitative Management Consultants, Inc.

Rizzolo, M. C., Hemp, R., Braddock, D., & Pomeranz-Essley, A.(2004). *The State of the States in Developmental Disabilities.* Washington, DC: American Association on Mental Retardation.

Statistical Abstracts of the United States, 2004-2005. Table 664. Http://www.census.gov/hhes/www/income.html

Stokes, T. F. & Baer, D. M. (1977). An implicit technology of generalization. *Journal of Applied Behavior Analysis, 10,* 349-67.

The Council on Quality and Leadership in Supports for People with Disabilities. *Personal Outcome Measures in Consumer-Directed Behavioral Health,* (2000). Towson, MD: Author.

Living Well with CMS Funding: A Study of Mortality in Wyoming

M. Chris Newman, M.H.A.; David J. Heath, M.P.A., Developmental Disabilities Division, Wyoming Department of Health; Jackie Olaveson, M.S.W., L.C.S.W., Wyoming Institute for Disabilities, University of Wyoming.

The natural life cycle of birth, growth, and death is unique to each individual. As professionals in the human services sector, we are interested in the risk factors that result in premature death and lifestyles that are associated with longevity. Among a dependent population such as persons with mental retardation and other developmental disabilities, lifestyle is partially dictated by the constraints of their residential setting and popular beliefs about the best setting in which their life cycle should be completed. Institutions were developed to provide appropriate treatment settings and to avoid the abuse and neglect that existed prior to their development. Institutional populations in many states are in decline due to litigation mainly because community placements are now seen as the preferred location for service provision to individuals with developmental disabilities.

Controversial research in California has suggested that placement into a community setting from an institution increases the risk of death (Strauss, Kastner, & Shavelle, 1998; Shavelle & Strauss, 1999) but there has been other research to refute that stance. It has been suggested by others (Blacher, 1998; Fujiura, 1998; Grossman & Eyman, 1998; Borthwick-Duffy, Widaaman, & Grossman, 1998) that comparisons between institutional and community placement are not focusing on the correct research question. Possible research could focus on: the factors of a quality life, accidents or abuse/neglect rates as well as natural deaths, and an analysis of appropriate health care as each relates to mortality rates. Given the research difficulty in controlling all variables in the institutional/community placement dichotomy, it certainly may benefit the field of developmental disabilities to focus on measurable factors that are related to mortality.

In the lead article of the October 1998 *Mental Retardation,* Hayden identifies common risk factors of mortality as age, level of mental retardation, non-ambulation, secondary medical conditions, presence of feeding tubes, and level of motor skills (p. 356). To this, we need to add the risk factor of community placement suggested by Strauss, et al. (1998) and Shavelle and Strauss (1999.) The contention that community placement constitutes a risk factor is not without controversy. O'Brien and Zaharia (1998) suggest that errors in the California data could account for the greater risk of mortality in community placements and that, when these errors are corrected, community placement would not be a risk factor. Conroy and Adler (1998) reviewed the records of persons placed into community settings from Pennhurst between 1978 and 1989, finding mortality rates that were lower than expected if the persons had remained at Pennhurst. Generally descriptive in nature, these studies should be reviewed with caution, for they do not adequately utilize controlled research design.

More recently, research on the subject of deinstitutionalization and mortality has sought to improve the research design. Lerman, Apgar, and Jordan (2003) matched a sample of 150 "movers" to 150 institutional "stayers" with the hope of being able to demonstrate differences between the community placement/institutional dichotomy using a more controlled research design. Lerman, Apgar, and Jordan found what others have found: it was not the placement in the community or the institution that determined the death rates but the specific risk factors for each individual that best explained who was most likely to die.

Wyoming's developmental disabilities system has received attention for developing progressive policies and procedures despite the fact that it is a profoundly rural state. Despite its small population, Wyoming has faced some of the same struggles that other states have weathered, such as deinstitutionalization. As was the case with institutions in California and Pennsylvania, the reduction in the census at Wyoming's lone institution, the Wyoming State Training School (WSTS), was the result of a class action lawsuit (*Weston, et al. v. Wyoming State Training School, et al.* C. 90-0004). However, unlike the Pennhurst case, *Weston* did not result in the closure of the institution. Between 1989 and present, WSTS populations decreased from 429 to the current census of 97 residents. Other than the obvious difference in the numbers of individuals involved (1,157 in Pennhurst and 22,576 in California), Wyoming is a frontier state, with sparse population and limited services in many areas, unlike California and Pennsylvania where there are decidedly larger populations and service sectors.

This effort is a continuation of our research into Wyoming's placement activity. Previous research has established that there were no significant differences between those who stayed at WSTS and those who moved in terms of the factors for mortality (level of mental retardation, adaptive behavior, maladaptive behavior, limitations on activities, and extent of medical care required [Heinlein & Fortune, 1995; Fortune, Heinlein, Fortune, 1995]). Mortality information in Wyoming is important to review, however, and, having a small sample size notwithstanding, we seek to find ways to analyze this information and improve the lives of those with developmental disabilities.

Method

Given a lack of sample size, we decided to take a different route with hopes of determining what risks, if any, are related to mortality for individuals with developmental disabilities. Combining individuals with developmental disabilities who reside in community placements with those who remain at the institution, there are only slightly over 1,000 total individuals. The small total number of individuals with developmental disabilities in Wyoming is directly related to the resulting small number of deaths (<200 since 1988).

The census of WSTS was 429 between 1989 and 1998. Of the total, 87 died, 133 remained at WSTS, and 209 have moved to settings other than WSTS. The 87 who died (31 died while at the WSTS, 56 died after placement) comprise the study population for the research done by Heinlein and Fortune.

In order to increase the data set totals, we added the total mortality counts of individuals receiving services from developmental disabilities services in Wyoming from 1988 to present. Information was gathered with regard to cause of death (as available), categorized, and analyzed for trends. Causes and dates of death were taken from the death certificates, Division of Developmental Disabilities incident reports, or service provider records, and were established for 134 individuals from 1988 to present. Those who have left the service system because of moving or dropping out have not been included in the count, and it is not known if they are living or dead.

Percentages of deaths for individuals with developmental disabilities from 1988 to present were compared to data provided by the Centers for Disease Control and Prevention (CDC), Department of Health and Human Services (2002) for all deaths in Wyoming and nationally. The CDC lists five chronic diseases that account for more than two-thirds of all deaths in the United States. These chronic diseases are:

- Heart Disease
- Cancers
- Stroke
- Chronic obstructive pulmonary diseases
- Diabetes

Data for the most common causes of death in the United States and Wyoming are contained in the tables 1 and 2.

Table 1

Most Common Causes of Death, United States, 1999*

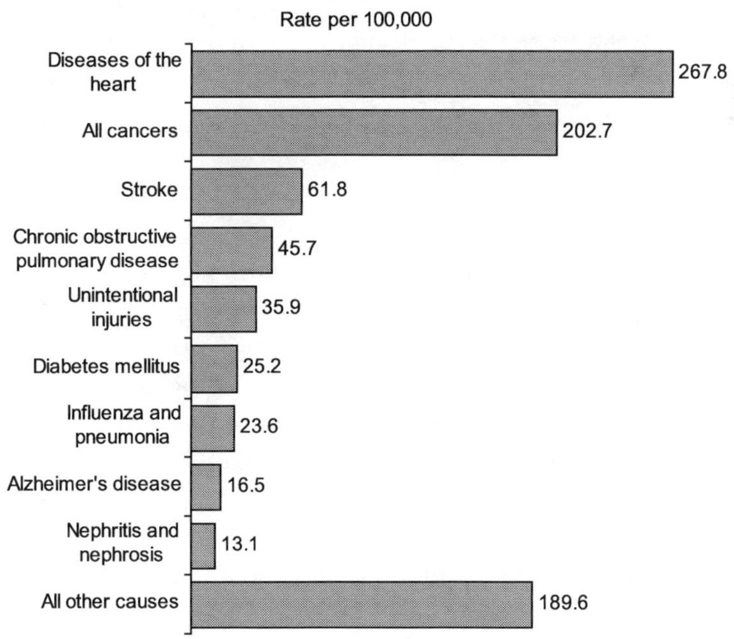

*Rates are age adjusted to 2000 total U.S. population.

CDC (2002)

Table 2
Causes of Death, Wyoming Compared with United States, 1999*

	Wyoming	United States
Diseases of the heart	231.1	267.8
All cancers	197.5	202.7
Stroke	61.7	61.8
Chronic obstructive pulmonary diseases	76.6	45.7
Unintentional injuries	53.8	35.9
Diabetes mellitus	30.1	25.2
Influenza and pneumonia	30.5	23.6
Alzheimer's disease	24.3	16.5
Nephritis and nephrosis	6.9	13.1
All other causes	196.2	189.6

*Deaths per 100,000, age adjusted to 2000 total U.S. population.
CDC (2002)

Heart disease, cancers, and stroke together account for almost 60% of all deaths in the United States. Of interest to the Wyoming DD system are those deaths that are attributable to causes that can be prevented or to those deaths that, with adequate health care, could be addressed to prolong the life of the individual. Percentages for the total deaths from 1988 to present for individuals with developmental disabilities were compared to the information for Wyoming and the United States as listed by the CDC (See Table 3).

Results

Within the limitation of the small total of the sample, there were some trends that bear mentioning for the figures noted in Table 3. There appear to be similarities in percentages in death rates for "diseases of the heart" and the "all others" categories when comparing the DD population death rates to the figures for the U.S. and Wyoming. The categories where the DD population death rates in Wyoming were higher than the U.S. and Wyoming's general population were "chronic respiratory disease" and the "influenza/pneumonia" categories. The "chronic respiratory disease" category was a little less than twice as high as that for the general Wyoming population, while the "influenza/pneumonia" percentages for the DD population were approximately three times higher than the general Wyoming population. Diseases of the kidney ("nephritis and nephrosis") as cause of death were also higher in Wyoming's DD population than the general population by about five times. “Stroke” was listed as the cause of death in only one case (0.7%) and the resulting percentage was much lower than that recorded for Wyoming’s general population (7.2%.) There were also no deaths recorded for “Alzheimer’s disease” or for “diabetes” in the DD population, but there are percentages for the general population of approximately 3.0% for both categories.

Table 3

	Wyoming + Adjusted per 100,000	Wyoming DD Population Deaths* (n=134)	United States + Adjusted per 100,000
Diseases of the heart	231.1 (27.0%)	41 (30.6%)	267.8 (29.0%)
All cancers	197.5 (23.1%)	11 (8.2%)	202.7 (22.9%)
Stroke	61.7 (7.2%)	1 (0.7)	61.8 (6.8%)
Chronic respiratory disease	76.6 (8.9%)	21 (15.7%)	45.7 (5.1%)
Diabetes	30.1 (3.5%)	0	25.2 (3.0%)
Influenza and pneumonia	30.5 (3.6%)	15 (11.2%)	23.6 (3.2%)
Alzheimer’s disease	24.3 (2.8%)	0	16.5 (2.3%)
Nephritis and nephrosis	6.9 (0.8%)	6 (4.5%)	13.1 (1.7%)
All others	196.2 (23.0%)	39 (29.1%)	189.6 (26.0%)
+ The Burden of Chronic Diseases and Their Risk Factors – 2002, Centers for Disease Control and Prevention, Department of Health and Human Services * All deaths since 1988			

The limitations in this information are inherent due to the diminutive number of deaths in the developmental disability population. With an average of less than nine deaths per year, there is little use in taking these numbers outside of Wyoming to make generalizations. There are, however, some interesting trends that were noted from the data. “Diseases of the respiratory system” and “influenza/pneumonia” as a cause of death were more common in the DD population by marked amounts and accounted for approximately one-fourth of the total DD deaths in Wyoming. It is likely that such diseases could be treated more effectively, thus decreasing death rates. With regard to diseases of the kidneys, it is also probable that the higher rates of mortality could also be treatable through increased wellness testing and early detection.

There certainly were flaws in collecting the details from the death certificates, which were mainly due to incomplete notations by physicians or coroners as to cause of death. There were no deaths attributable to diabetes or Alzheimer’s disease in Wyoming’s DD population despite evidence of both diseases on a national and state level. These two diseases were not listed as secondary or tertiary on any of the death records reviewed. It is known that there were deaths of several individuals who had Down syndrome and had Alzheimer-like symptoms. However, the death certificates did not list Alzheimer dementia but some other cause of death, such as pneumonia. There also were many certificates that had vague classifications of death, such as "multi-system failure" or "death from natural causes" that could be attributable to a more specific category, but were instead listed in the category of "All Others." The problem here is not with the DD service system, but the method by which death certificates are completed. Many of the death certificates had primary, secondary, and tertiary causes of death listed and as such, had very definable causality for death. If the primary cause of death was listed as coronary failure but the secondary and tertiary causes were defined as respiratory disease, the cause of death was listed as respiratory in nature because that condition led to the failure of the heart function.

Discussion

It would undoubtedly be helpful to examine the reasons for risk, analyze health care practices as they relate to mortality, and investigate what determines mortality. While this study is descriptive in nature, it is hoped that outcomes will yield direction for further research on the factors for mortality in Wyoming specifically by guiding research toward an analysis of the factors that can be influenced by the State Developmental Disabilities personnel, providers of services, family members, and self-advocates. There are higher death rates for diseases of the lungs (respiratory disease and influenza/pneumonia) and the kidney (nephritis and nephrosis) than in the general population of Wyoming. Could the health care of individuals with developmental disabilities be focused on these factors and would such an effort demonstrate decreases in death rates? It is difficult to generalize these results, even within Wyoming. Given the profound rural status of Wyoming and the size of the data set, there are also obvious difficulties in generalizing results to other states. Nancy Thaler, Director for Quality Improvement Strategies for Home and Community Based Services of the Centers for Medicare and Medicaid Services in Baltimore, felt that this paper is an excellent example of a state dealing with practical risk management at a statewide level.

It has been difficult to gather accurate data, but with new reporting procedures and increased communication from Division staff, the foundation is in place for more accurate recording of mortality rates. It is also difficult to take information from such a small section of individuals and make reliable generalizations. Despite the drawbacks for generalization, analysis should continue, for with its small population and outstanding service system Wyoming stands to make great strides towards decreasing preventable mortality and improving quality of life for individuals with developmental disabilities. With the hope of yielding a higher quality of life through increased longevity for persons with developmental disabilities, future research and analysis could be focused on:

1. Improving health care through more thorough preventive measures
   - Recent data collection through Core Indicators Wyoming on physicals and OB/GYN exams is encouraging. The rates of physicals and other exams have increased each year that the data have been collected.
   - Encouraging providers of DD services to improve the scheduling of routine health care through the use of computerized data tracking systems

2. Increasing longevity of those with developmental disabilities
   - Identifying preventable injuries and illnesses early and providing adequate health care when identified

3. Refining and improving the reporting mechanisms for deaths and other risk factors
   - Reviewing death certificates for complete information

4. Comparison of mortality trends and rates for those with developmental disabilities and those in the general population
   - Analysis of quality of life factors, i.e., rate of annual physicals, causes of mortality, death from abuse/neglect, nutrition, etc. in relation to deaths
   - Analysis of rates of the type of mortality and how such rates relate to preventable or postponable factors

5. Analyzing levels and types of service in relation to mortality for trends

6. Analysis of community supports with regard to healthcare, specifically with regard to rural settings and lack of adequate health care services and professionals in small towns

In addition, the Wyoming Developmental Disabilities Division has established a process for reviewing deaths of persons served to identify trends and assure that the appropriate services and supports were provided. Below is a summary of the committee processes, including membership, case review, and data collection and analysis.

Mortality Review Committee Membership

The Committee includes the following:

- Program Integrity Manager, chairperson
- Physician
- Program Integrity Nurse
- Waiver Managers
- Area Resource Specialist
- Survey/Certification QMRP

Case Review

The Committee will meet twice a year, in January and July, to review the deaths that have occurred during the previous six-month period. July's meeting will review deaths that have occurred between January and June of the calendar year and January's meeting will include a review of deaths that occur between July and December of the previous calendar year. The first meeting is scheduled for July 2005.

The following material will be distributed to the committee before each meeting:

- Copy of current plan of care for person served
- Copy of all incident reports for person served for past 12 months, including incident report notifying the Division of the death
- Copies of results of Division visits/interviews or team meeting notes with person served family, guardian or staff for the past 12 month period if applicable
- Copy of coroner's report if applicable.
- Copy of provider documentation if questions/concerns are noted surrounding death.
- Summary of total number of deaths for current time period and aggregate information on all deaths for past three years.
- Results of evaluation of deaths by cause of death, provider, waiver, age and other pertinent analyses.

Database

The Division will maintain a database that summarizes pertinent information on the deaths, including:

- Age at time of death
- Gender
- Cause of death
- Diagnoses
- Residential provider
- Where death occurred
- Waiver

Recommendations of the Committee

The committee can make recommendations based on the review of the deaths. Recommendations can be provider specific or systemic. Recommendations that are provider specific must tie directly to current rules, recommendations or standards that are in place. Program Integrity will review provider specific recommendations and follow-up with providers. Systemic recommendations will be forwarded to the Division's management committee for review and, when appropriate, implementation. Recommendations will be tracked to assure they are reviewed and addressed when appropriate.

References

Blacher, J. (1998). The California mortality controversy: Much ado about mortality: Debating the wrong question. *Mental Retardation, 36,* 412-415.

Borthwick-Duffy, S., Widaman, K., & Grossman, H. (1998). Mortality research, placement, and risk of death: Basic research, the media, and public policy. *Mental Retardation, 36,* 416-422.

Conroy, J. W. & Adler, M. (1998). Mortality among Pennhurst class members, 1978 to 1989: A brief report. *Mental Retardation, 36,* 380-385.

Fortune, J., Heinlein, K. B., & Fortune, B. (1995). Changing the shape of the service population. *European Journal on Mental Disabilities, 2,* 20-37

Fujiura, G. T. (1998). Commentary on the meaning of residential mortality research. *Mental Retardation, 36,* 400-402.

Grossman, H. & Eyman, R., Historical perspective on mortality and placement. *Mental Retardation, 36,* 237-239.

Hayden, M. F. (1998). Mortality among people with mental retardation living in the United States: Research and policy applications. *Mental Retardation, 36,* 345-359.

Heinlein, K. B. & Fortune, J. (1995). Who stays, who goes? Downsizing the institution in America's most rural state. *Research in Developmental Disabilities, 16,* 165-177.

Lerman, P., Apgar, D. H., & Jordan, T. (2003). Deinstitutionalization and mortality: Findings of a controlled research design in New Jersey. *Mental Retardation, 41,* 225-236.

O'Brien, K. F. & Zaharia, E. S. (1998). Recent mortality patterns in California. *Mental Retardation, 36,* 372-379.

Shavelle, R. & Strauss, D. (1999). Mortality of persons with developmental disabilities after transfer into community care: A 1996 update. *American Journal on Mental Retardation, 104,* 143-147.

Strauss, D., Kastner, T. A., & Shavelle, R. (1998). Mortality of adults with developmental disabilities living in California institutions and community care, 1985-1994. *Mental Retardation, 36,* 360-379.

Fiscal Issues

Predicting Individual Budgets in a Support Program for People with Developmental Disabilities: An Evaluation

Edward A. Konarski, Jr., Human Development Research and Training Institute at J. Iverson Riddle Developmental Center; Rodney E. Realon, North Carolina Division of Mental Health/Developmental Disabilities/Substance Abuse Services; Marc J. Tassé, Center for Development and Learning, University of North Carolina at Chapel Hill

Introduction

The purpose of this research was to evaluate the usefulness of a statistical method for predicting individual budgets for consumers in publicly administered support programs for people with developmental disabilities. Ed Campbell and his colleagues pioneered this methodology for use in this area (e.g., Campbell, 2002; Campbell & Heal, 1995; Campbell et al., 2005). Their approach is based on the premise that differences in cost of service to people with developmental disabilities living in community settings can be accounted for by differences in individual needs for supports and other quantifiable factors that can be determined through systematic analysis (Fortune et al., 2005). They use the statistical method of multiple regression to identify the variables that contribute to differences in cost. This statistical technique can select, from the variety of variables submitted for analysis, those that make a significant contribution to predicting a particular outcome. In the present case, the particular outcome of interest is the yearly cost of service for an individual consumer. The outcome of this analysis is a mathematical formula that can predict a portion of the variance in cost of service delivery for individual consumers in a particular service system. From the variables entered into the analysis, the resulting formula reflects only those variables that make an independent contribution to predicting cost. Furthermore, the formula includes the weighting for each variable that reflects the relative importance of their contribution to predicting financial cost of support.

Campbell and his colleagues have presented several analyses using their approach for predicting individual budgets for people with developmental disabilities and found that it can account for 52% to as much as 88% of the variability in actual program costs among consumers (Campbell, Fortune, & Severance, 2000; Fortune et al., 2005). While this approach is not able to account for all of the variability in costs among consumers, this degree of predictive power makes this a potentially valuable approach for understanding, establishing, and actively managing individual budgets for people with developmental disabilities accessing publicly managed programs that support their service needs. It also provides a systematic methodology for establishing budgets for individuals that focuses on quantitative and objective measures that will help insure that people are receiving financial support commensurate with their particular service situation. Hence, we sought to use this approach in the North Carolina Community Alternative Program (CAP MR/DD) to determine how effective it would be in accounting for individual yearly costs.

This approach for predicting yearly program costs would seem to have great value for consumers and administrators alike. For example, in the 2001-2002 budget year, North Carolina had to address a budget shortfall of about $1.6 billion dollars in its general budget. This was an astounding amount given that the state budget was approximately $14.3 billion dollars. Such a situation mandates that government look for strategies to fairly and equitably allocate its limited resources. It would seem that an objective approach based on a standardized procedure such as multiple regression that identifies the variability in consumer costs would assist in this allocation of financial resources. This approach has the merit of attempting to equitably distribute resources based on individual characteristics and support needs. Additionally, with many states having long waiting lists for services, this approach provides a potential tool for providing legislators and administrators with an objective means of knowing how resources can concretely reduce these long waiting lists. Individuals from the advocacy field are also excited by this work since the ability to precisely estimate individualized budgets is a natural precursor to portability of budgets (Fortune et al., 2005).

From the perspective of consumers and their family, knowing what resources are available can reduce the anxiety associated with trying to put together an array of services to meet the diverse and sometimes complex needs identified in a person centered plan. An objective approach to budget allocation would seem to be of assistance in this process by reducing uncertainty regarding the method for establishing financial resources.

In the present analysis, we applied the techniques of multiple regression similarly to Campbell and his colleagues to analyze the data in the North Carolina CAP MR/DD Program . The CAP MR/DD program arose out of federal legislation in the form of Medicaid that was passed as Title XIX of the Social Security Act (PL 89-97). Medicaid is an entitlement program meaning that persons who are eligible have a legal right to services offered under this program. While initially designed to meet the health needs of low-income elderly persons, the Medicaid program has evolved to also meet the long term care needs of persons with developmental disabilities. The CAP MR/DD program is a home and community based services waiver that falls under this legislation. We were seeking to develop a statistical model that would predict the yearly cost of care for program participants so that we might evaluate its accuracy and consider its value as the basis for establishing individual budgets.

Method for Developing the Model

Variables Entered

The variables entered into the analysis developed by Campbell and his colleagues came from information existing in databases typically maintained by states in providing services to people with developmental disabilities (Campbell, 2002; Campbell & Heal, 1995; Campbell et al., 2005). These included such variables as recent past costs for services for individual consumers, individual consumer services utilization, consumer demographic information, local geographic and economic data, and, a measure of consumer need for service. We were unable to utilize the identical set of variables used by Campbell and his colleagues because of the differences between the state systems. However, we did use readily available variables, many of which closely match those in their studies. The variables used in the present analyses were obtained from existing North Carolina CAP MR/DD databases. All information was obtained through the support of the North Carolina Developmental Disabilities Section, the state agency that oversees this program.

The specific dependent variable of interest (i.e., the predicted variable) in this study was the total amount of CAP MR/DD funds allocated to an individual consumer for the entire fiscal year. A total of 47 independent (predictor) variables were entered into the multiple regression analysis with the intent of establishing a formula to predict cost of services for individuals in the CAP MR/DD program. The particular variables that were used are listed in Table 1. All data used was from the 2001 fiscal year.

Consumer Support Need

Campbell and his group have employed the *Inventory for Client and Agency Planning* (*ICAP*– Bruininks, Hill, Weatherman, & Woodcock, 1986) as a standardized measure of the extent of consumer need for supports. Unfortunately, North Carolina does not use this particular assessment measure so it was not available in existing data sources. However, in order to assess this critical variable of cost analysis, in this study the extent of support need for each consumer was determined using the *North Carolina Support Needs Assessment Profile* (*NCSNAP*). The instrument consists of 11 questions that are divided into three domains (Daily Living Supports, Health Care Supports, and Behavioral Supports). Scoring is based on 5 levels with 1 indicating the least amount of supports and 5 representing the highest level of supports. For each domain, the highest score indicated for an item represents the level of need for that domain. An overall level is determined by taking the highest level among the three domains. This assessment has been used in North Carolina since 1999.

Consumers

There were 6,194 participants in the North Carolina CAP MR/DD program during the 2001 fiscal year. Participants not in the program for the entire year or whose dataset was incomplete were eliminated from the study. This resulted in a total of 3,201 participants in the original database developed for this study. Another 271 participants were eliminated from this group prior to our analysis because it was noted that they also received significant funding from other program sources in addition to the CAP MR/DD program of interest in this study. Therefore, the initial multiple regression analysis to develop the predictive model was run with the data of 2,930 consumers from the North Carolina CAP MR/DD program. This

Table 1
Predictor Variables entered into Multiple Regression Analysis*

Support Need
1) SNAP Level
2) SNAP Raw Score
3) SNAP Index Score
4) SNAP Domain Score
5) SNAP Daily Living Domain Score
6) SNAP Health Care Domain Score
7) SNAP Behavioral Supports Domain Score

Demographic Information
8) Residential Placement
9) Age
10) Gender
11) Race
12) Level of Mental Retardation

Other Measures
13) Area Program
14) % Poverty in County
15) County Census
16) County Income Level
17) Rating of Service Appropriateness
18) CAP Units
19) LOS Axis 1
20) LOS Axis 2
21) LOS Axis 3
22) LOS Axis 4
23) Autism

CAP Services Utilized (Yes/No)
24) Community Inclusion – Group
25) Community Inclusion – Individual
26) Day Habilitation – Group 2
27) Day Habilitation – Group 3
28) Day Habilitation – Individual
29) Developmental Day Program
30) Durable Medical Equipment
31) Home Health
32) Inpatient General Hospital
33) Mental Retardation - Personal Care
34) Mental Retaration - Waiver Supplies
35) Outpatient General Hospital
36) Non Physician Services
37) Prescription Drugs
38) Prevocational Services – Group 1
39) Prevocational Services – Group 2
40) Prevocational Services – Individual
41) Respite - Individual
42) Respite – Group Home
43) Respite – Nursing Home
44) Supported Employment Services
45) Supervised Living
46) Supported Living
47) Physician Services

represents 47.3% of the total number of participants in the program during the fiscal year of this study. The mean age of the participants was 25.9 years (range = 4 – 78 years). Fifty-eight percent were male while 42% were female. Regarding race, 67% were Caucasian, 28.3% were African-American, and 4.2% were listed as other races. Looking at level of mental retardation, 13.3% were in the mild range of mental retardation, 30.8% in the moderate range, 28.6% in the severe range, and 22.6% in the profound range. The remainder were listed as unknown. The percentage of people at each of the 5 levels of support need indicated on the *NC-SNAP* were .2% at Level 1 (lowest level of support need), 3.9% at Level 2, 44.7% at Level 3, 41.9% at Level 4, and 9.2% at Level 5 (highest level of support need).

Statistical Method

The particular multiple regression approach used by Campbell and his colleagues for predicting individual cost of service is called stepwise linear multiple regression. Using this method, predictions of cost (dependent variable) can be made by considering several variables simultaneously (independent or predictor variables). The outcome of this analysis is a linear equation containing the variables that produce the least mathematical distance from the line that best describes the observed scores on the dependent variable. Each of these variables in the equation is assigned a weight that reflects its relative contribution in the final equation and its relationship relative to the dependent variable. This is a relatively common statistical technique that is utilized in a variety of settings where it is known that more than one variable influences the outcome on a measure and where there is interest in predicting a specific outcome.

This approach considers all variability in a set of data; therefore, the proportion of variability in cost accounted for by each component of the equation can be determined. This measure is called R^2 (R squared) and the sum of this statistic for each of the variables in the regression equation gives the total amount of variability accounted for in the set of data regarding the predicted variable (i.e., individual yearly cost of care). In a perfect model, all variables influencing the predicted variable would be included and thus permit the ability to explain 100% of the variability in yearly cost to consumers. The sum of the amount of variability accounted for is important in the present case because it is an estimate of the degree to which the equation can accurately predict yearly cost of care. This total R^2 sum can vary between 0.0 and 1.0 (where 1.0 represents 100% of the variability accounted for) and the closer to 1.0, the greater the predictive value, or accuracy, of the model. As mentioned, Campbell and his colleagues report that they were able to account for as much as .88, or 88% of the variability in program costs in their analyses (Campbell, et al., 2000). In the social sciences, this is most definitely a significant figure. The amount of variability in cost that is not accounted for by the equation is determined by subtracting the known variability from 1.0 and is referred to as error for the sources of this variability are unknown. This error might likely be reduced in the present approach by adding additional variables to the model which could explain more variability in annual costs, or perhaps by improving the accuracy of existing variables. Either way, researchers have potential avenues for gaining a greater understanding of the variables that account for costs in their system of supports.

Creating the Model

The 47 variables were entered into a stepwise multiple linear regression analysis with yearly cost of care per consumer as the dependent variable. The resulting statistical model is presented in Table 2. The variables are listed in order of greatest contribution of variability to predicting yearly cost. The column "Multiple R" shows the correlation of the model with yearly cost at that step of the analysis. The column "Multiple R^2" shows the squared correlation, which is the measure of the amount of variability in cost that the model cumulatively can account for at that step. The "Change in R^2" column lists the amount of variability added to the model at that particular step. The "F to enter" column displays the F statistic which tests the significance of the simple linear regression between that variable and yearly cost at that step of the analysis.

Table 2
Initial Statistical Model of Yearly Cost per Consumer

Variable	Multiple R	Multiple R^2	Change in R^2	F to Enter
CAP units	0.5272	0.2779	0.2779	1126.99
Supported Living	0.6507	0.4234	0.1455	738.52
Residential Placement	0.7276	0.5294	0.1060	659.12
Prevocational – Individual	0.7487	0.5605	0.0311	207.16
Community Inclusion – Individual	0.7648	0.5849	0.0244	171.58
Supported Employment – Indiv.	0.7767	0.6033	0.0184	135.32
Age	0.7850	0.6162	0.0129	98.22
Community Inclusion – Group	0.7879	0.6208	0.0047	35.96
Prevocational Services – Group 2	0.7904	0.6247	0.0039	30.26
County Census	0.7920	0.6272	0.0025	19.72
Day Habilitation – Individual	0.7933	0.6293	0.0021	16.57
Mental Retardation Personal Care	0.7942	0.6308	0.0015	11.71
Prescription Drugs	0.7950	0.6321	0.0013	9.99
Inpatient General Hospital	0.7958	0.6332	0.0011	9.04
Gender	0.7963	0.6341	0.0009	6.95
Level of Mental Retardation	0.7968	0.6349	0.0008	6.72
Physician Services	0.7973	0.6357	0.0008	6.04
County Income Level	0.7977	0.6364	0.0007	5.38
Home Health	0.7981	0.6370	0.0006	5.00

This model contains 19 of the 47 variables that were entered into the analysis for predicting yearly cost per consumer. Looking at the last figure in the "Multiple R^2" column, it can be seen that this statistical model is able to account for approximately 64% of the variability that goes into determining yearly cost of care for consumers in this funding program. Looking at the "Change in R^2" column it is obvious that the combination of the first three variables of CAP units, supported living, and residential placement account for the largest share of variability (53%) while the remaining 16 factors account for a relatively small amount of variability (11%) in yearly costs.

In order to refine this model, we eliminated from further analysis those cases where the model was unable to provide a reasonable prediction of actual costs. It was decided that those cases where the difference between actual cost and cost predicted by the model was greater than 3 standard deviations from the average of this difference would be classified as an outlier and removed from analysis (Campbell, 2002). This difference between actual and predicted cost is referred to as the residual cost. This is an important statistic in determining the viability of a regression model for it assesses exactly how accurate the model is in predicting outcomes. Therefore, those cases where the model does not produce a reasonable estimate of costs represent a failure of the model. Low residual costs indicate that the costs predicted by the model closely match the actual costs incurred by the consumer while high residual costs suggest that the model is predicting yearly costs very different from actual costs. In examining the predicted vs. the actual costs for each case using this model, 18 cases were found to exceed the cutoff of 3 standard deviations from the average residual. These cases were eliminated and the multiple regression analysis was re-run using only the remaining cases. This process of developing a model for predicting costs and eliminating outliers based on the predictions of the model was repeated until a model resulted where no outliers could be identified according to our criterion of a residual cost greater than 3 standard deviations from the mean residual cost A total of 6 models were developed in this process of model refinement and a total of 29 individual cases were eliminated as outliers resulting in a final model that used a sample size of 2,901 (2,930 original cases less the 29 outliers identified through the development of the six statistical models). Our criterion for identifying outliers resulted in less than 1% of the participants being removed from the process of model development.

Table 3
Final Statistical Model of Yearly Cost per Consumer

Variable	Multiple R	Multiple R^2	Change in R^2	F to Enter
CAP units	0.5265	0.2772	0.2772	1112.03
Supported Living	0.6626	0.4391	0.1618	836.12
Residential Placement	0.7434	0.5526	0.1136	735.47
Prevocational. – Individual	0.7654	0.5858	0.033123	1.77
Community Inclusion – Individual	0.7831	0.6133	0.0275	205.50
Supported Employment. – Ind.	0.7960	0.6337	0.0204	161.18
Age	0.8045	0.6472	0.0135	110.96
Community Inclusion -Group	0.8071	0.6514	0.0042	34.74
Prevocational Services – Group 2	0.8093	0.6549	0.0036	29.92
Mental Retardation Personal Care	0.8120	0.6594	0.0045	37.90
County Census	0.8132	0.6613	0.0019	16.43
Day Habilitation – Individual	0.8143	0.6631	0.0018	15.50
Physician	0.8152	0.6646	0.0015	12.62
Level of Mental Retardation	0.8160	0.6659	0.0013	11.38
Inpatient General Hospital	0.8167	0.6670	0.0010	8.98
Gender	0.8173	0.6679	0.0010	8.44
SNAP Behavior Support Domain	0.8178	0.6688	0.0008	7.25
County Income Level	0.8182	0.6694	0.0006	5.49
Men. Retardation Waiver Supplies	0.8185	0.6699	0.0005	4.57
Home Health	0.8189	0.6705	0.0006	5.23

The components of this final model are presented in Table 3 which is structured exactly as Table 2. It can be seen that the model contains 20 variables, not all of which are identical to those in the initial model. As outliers were eliminated from the analysis the components of the initial model and their contributions to variability in yearly consumer cost were altered. This final model was able to predict yearly consumer costs that were within 3 standard deviations of the average residual cost for each of the cases. It also was able to account for slightly more variability in the yearly cost data than the initial model as total R^2 for this final model was slightly over 67%. The total variability accounted for by this final model compares favorably with that of Campbell and his colleagues who reported total variability accounted for of between 52 and 88% in their various analyses. As in the initial model, the variables of CAP units, supported living, and residential placement accounted for the majority of the known variability (55%) while the remaining 17 variables accounted for the remaining 12%.

The fact that little variability in costs is actually contributed by the 17 variables at the bottom of the list might suggest that inclusion of these variables could be an example of "over fitting," that is, including unnecessary variables in the model. However, the tolerances for each of the variables in the final model far exceeded the criterion of .20 utilized by Campbell and his colleagues (Campbell et al., 2005). In fact, none of the variables in our final model had tolerances of less than .50. Tolerances above this level suggest that each of these variables is likely contributing an independent source of variability. Therefore, in order to maximize the predictive power of the model, all variables identified were maintained as part of the model.

Finally, an important issue in using multiple linear regression is the number of cases studied in relation to the number of variables entered into the analysis. One rule states that there must be at least 50 cases for each predictor variable entered into the analysis when developing the model. In this study, 47 variables were entered into analysis; therefore, there should be at least 2,350 cases for study (47 x 50). Another rule states that the number of cases used must be greater than 50 + 8 times the number of variables entered into the analysis. In this case, that would mean at least 426 cases (50 + 8 x 47) should be used. The number of cases actually used in this study is 2,901, thereby easily exceeding accepted standards for using multiple linear regression (Cohen, 1988).

In summary, we have developed a model for predicting individual yearly budgets in the North Carolina CAP MR/DD program. The model was developed using the statistical approach of stepwise linear multiple regression following the example of Campbell and his colleagues. All of the variables used as predictors of yearly cost were readily available in the existing state data systems and approximated those used by Campbell and his colleagues. A total of 47 predictor variables were entered into the analysis. The final model developed contains 20 of these variables and is able to account for approximately 67% of the variability in yearly costs which compares favorably with earlier work. Tolerance checks suggest that each variable in the final model contributes an independent source of variability in yearly costs. Furthermore, the number of cases included in model development exceeds the amount required for meeting acceptable standards in applying the technique of multiple regression. Therefore, we believe that we have produced an acceptable model for predicting yearly consumer costs in the program studied. We will now turn to our evaluation of this model for predicting individual budgets.

Evaluating the Model

Evaluation 1

At the start, we must note that actual budgets for consumers in the North Carolina CAP MR/DD Program were calculated and implemented independent of all of our analyses. The evaluations presented here use historical data to note the possible impact of the approach that we are taking to developing individual budgets so that it might be considered for future use.

A simple method to evaluate the model developed in this analysis is to compare costs predicted by the model with those actually incurred by the consumers in the sample used to develop the model. As mentioned above, the difference between these two costs is called the residual cost (residual cost = actual cost - predicted cost). When the predicted cost for a consumer is less than his/her actual cost, this is referred to as under prediction and is reflected as a positive residual cost. When the predicted cost for a consumer is greater than his/her actual cost, this is referred to as over prediction and is reflected as a negative residual cost.

Figure 1

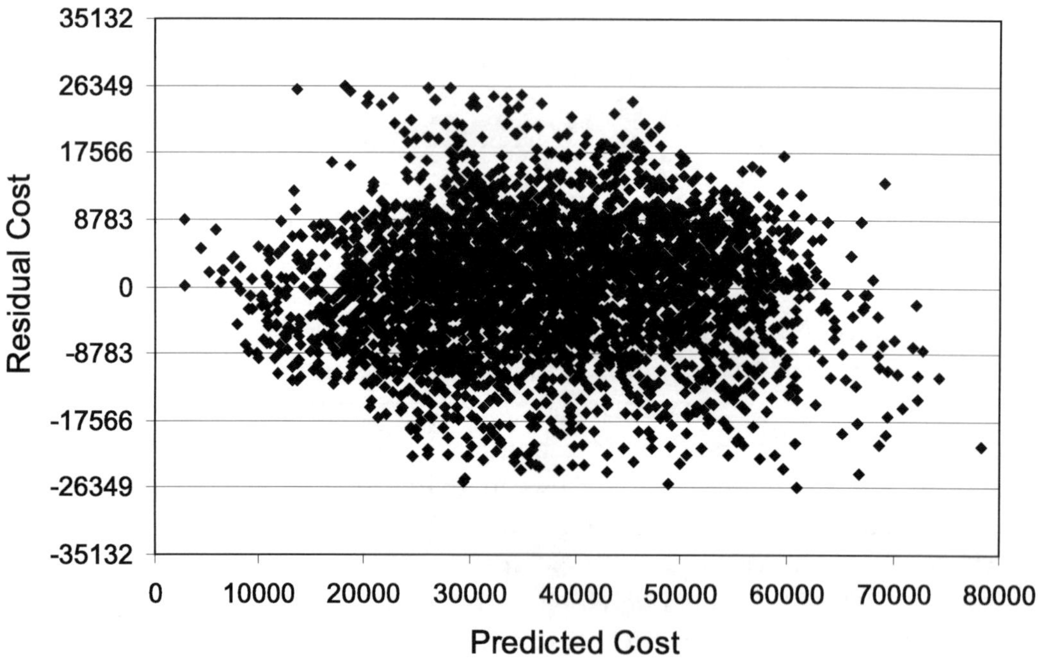

Figure 1 depicts the residual costs for each of the cases included in the final model (N = 2901). In this figure, the predicted costs are on the x axis and the residual on the y axis. The more accurate the model, the more residual costs will cluster along the gridline indicating 0 on the y axis (an exact match of predicted and actual costs). Each gridline represents one standard deviation ($8,783) of residual costs. As one would expect, it can readily be seen that the vast majority of the residuals clustered within 1 standard deviation of 0. Relatively few residuals were greater than 2 standard deviations from 0. This was true across the range of predicted costs, although errors appear more likely at either extreme. Specifically, there appears to be a tendency for the model to under predict actual cost for individuals at the lower level of predicted spending (upper left quadrant of figure 1) and to over predict costs for individuals at the higher end of predicted spending (lower right quadrant of figure 1). Overall, the pattern of residual costs created by these data indicate that the model does a respectable job of predicting yearly costs as the residual costs remain relatively close to 0 across all of the values of predicted costs. If the pattern of residual costs was more scattered in this figure, it would indicate that the model does a poor job of predicting costs that approximate actual costs for consumers. It should be noted that this analysis is not a strong assessment of the predictive validity of the model as the actual costs to consumers was the dependent variable used to develop the model for generating the predicted costs.

We examined the size of the residuals closely as they reflect the real world differences between the amount that an individual would be budgeted if this approach were used to develop individual budgets and what they actually spent in fiscal 2001. We found that 259 individuals (8.9% of the sample) had residuals with an absolute value greater than $15,000. Since the average yearly consumer cost was $37,752, this seems like a significant error in prediction. Thus, based on this evaluation we would expect that the predicted individual budget for approximately 91% of persons would fall reasonably close to their actual annual budgets. Conversely, some sort of budgetary correction would be needed for at least 9% of individuals.

Evaluation 2

A more stringent test of the final model developed for predicting cost in the North Carolina CAP MR/DD Program is to use the model to predict costs for people who were not in the sample on which the model was developed. We were able to accomplish this test by finding 373 additional cases from the 2001 fiscal year which were not included in the original sample. The model was used to predict the costs of these individuals and the results were compared to the actual costs for this independent sample of consumers. The results are depicted in Figure 2 and it is set up exactly as Figure 1, with predicted costs on the x axis and the residual costs, or difference from actual cost, on the y axis. Gridlines once again represent one standard deviation ($10,516).

Figure 2

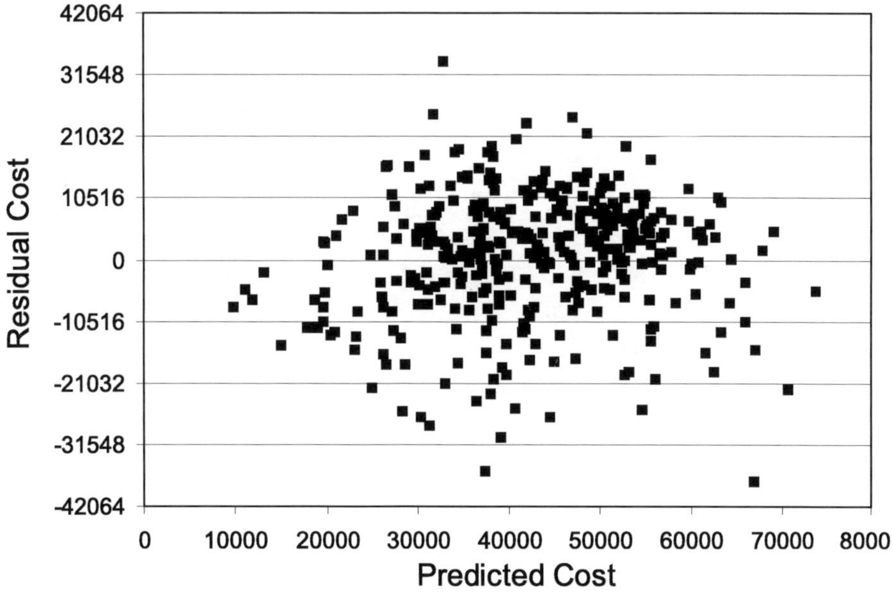

It can be seen that residuals clearly clustered around the 0 gridline indicating no difference between actual and predicted costs and the large majority of residuals were within 1 standard deviation. While there are some residuals that are as many as 3 standard deviations from 0, these are clearly a very small percentage of the sample (< 1%). The spread of scores differs slightly from that seen in Evaluation 1 for the only obvious tendency in this analysis is that the model tended to over predict scores at the higher end of predicted costs (lower right quadrant of figure). The mean predicted cost for the consumers in this analysis is $42,261 while their actual cost has a mean of $43,000, reflecting a small ($739), non-statistically significant difference (t = .476, df = 372). Therefore, it appears that while the model under predicts cost by about $739 per person (< 2% of actual budget), it nonetheless does a good job of predicting actual individual consumer costs when evaluating all of the predicted costs as a group. However, it is easily noted by looking at Figure 2 that the model poorly predicted yearly consumer cost for a number of people as some residuals exceeded $23,000, more than half of mean per consumer actual costs. As in Evaluation 1, we counted all individuals whose residuals had an absolute value greater than $15,000 and found that 51 people exceeded this criterion (13.7% of sample).

Evaluation 3

An even more stringent, and perhaps the most practical, evaluation of the validity of the final model for predicting individual budgets developed in this project would be to compare the predictions of the model against the actual costs of the consumers in the following fiscal year (i.e., FY 2002). This would be an application of one of the potential uses of the model, which is using the data from the prior fiscal year to predict costs for the subsequent year. If the model is able to produce a reasonable prediction of actual costs in a subsequent year, it would seem to have value for managers in attempting to predict future program costs, and, for individuals in budgeting to meet the needs of their person centered plan. To do this, the individual costs and relevant program data utilized by the model for the consumers in the 2002 fiscal year were obtained from the State Section of Developmental Disabilities. A total of 2,858 of the 2,901 consumers that were in the original sample in 2001 were also in the CAP MR/DD program for the full year of 2002 and had records that included updated data on the variables that were used to calculate predicted cost. Using the final model developed on the data of 2001, predicted costs were calculated for 2002. The comparison of these predicted costs with the actual costs incurred by the consumers in 2002 is shown in Figure 3.

It can be clearly seen that the vast majority of residuals were concentrated around the gridline indicating no difference between predicted and actual costs for the fiscal year 2002. Once again, there appears to be a tendency for the model to over predict costs at the upper level of predicted costs (lower right quadrant) and under predict costs at the lower level of predicted costs (upper left quadrant). Nonetheless, the concentration of residuals around 0 suggests that the model does an adequate job of predicting costs under the practical circumstances of this particular evaluation. The mean residual was $3,648, suggesting an overall under prediction of actual costs as was found in Evaluation 2. It should be noted that this mean residual was much larger than that seen when the model developed using 2001 data was used with the data of other consumers from that year who were not in the dataset used to develop the model. In 2001, the mean residual was only $739. Therefore, the predictive validity of the model when applied to a subsequent year would appear to be much less than when it is applied to consumers within the same year, even when their data was not part of model development.

Figure 3

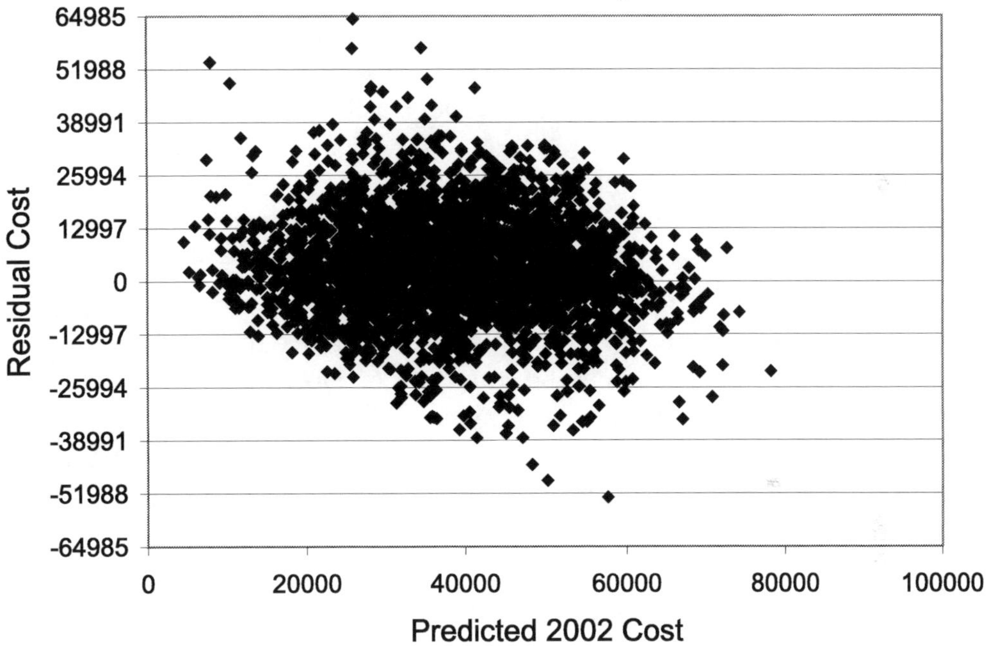

Examining Figure 3, it can be seen that there were some cases where the model made very poor predictions, with some residuals greater than $50,000! Again we counted the number of cases where residuals had an absolute value greater than $15,000 and found 647 such cases. This represents 22.6% of the sample in this study.

Evaluation 4

In another test of the predictive validity of the final model developed in this study, also using the 2002 cost data, the residuals from Evaluation 3 were compared to those which resulted when the actual 2002 costs were compared to the consumers' 2001 actual costs. In essence, the predictions of the model were compared to using the prior year's cost as the predicted cost for the next year. As noted above, the mean of the residuals for the model's predictions in Evaluation 3 was \$3,648 while the mean of the residuals found when using 2001's cost to predict 2002 cost was \$3,551. This is a small (\$97) and non-statistically significant difference ($t = .59328$; $df = 2857$). It is also interesting to note that 486 individuals (17%) had a residual with an absolute value greater than \$15,000, which is 161 fewer than found when using the model to predict costs. These outcomes suggest that the use of a model developed through linear multiple regression to predict costs in the next year may not be superior to simply using a person's prior year cost data to predict cost in the next year.

Limitations of this Analysis

As with any research effort, there are some limitations that must be noted in order to best evaluate the outcomes. First, this analysis only looks at one specific population of consumers with developmental disabilities served by the state of North Carolina. Therefore, the specific model developed here is appropriate only for this population and cannot be generalized for use with other populations served or with similar populations in other States. That said, models can be developed for individuals in other service groups (e.g., Dual Diagnosis, ICF-MR, etc.) and/or in other states using this same approach, given the appropriate data.

Second, with the statistical approach used, an individual's budget is predicted from the averages of many people and may not reflect that individual exactly. Therefore, there will almost always be some degree of error in predicting precise individual budgets. This error may not be significant when evaluating an overall program budget as over predictions and under predictions by the model will tend to balance out and hence, overall program costs will be relatively accurate as the research presented here has demonstrated. However, this error is an especially important factor to consider when using the approach to develop individual budgets since our evaluations show that in some cases there will be a large difference between predicted costs and the actual costs incurred by a consumer. This finding suggests the need for a mechanism to mediate individual cases where the predicted budget is discrepant with actual consumer support needs. The very nature of the technique of multiple regression for predicting individual budgets will result in some people being allotted more than might be expected while others will be allotted less as the mathematical procedures work to reduce the distance of all cases from the best fit line of a set of data. We noted some of these significant discrepancies in our evaluations.

Third, this approach uses historical data to guide the future. This can become problematic when changes occur in consumers or in the service delivery system which influence individual costs. While some changes can be accounted for such as a planned change in reimbursement rates, other changes such as a sudden increase or decrease in the availability of a support service, unexpected consumer medical complications, or rapid economic shifts cannot be anticipated by the model. The model is clearly most accurate in a relatively stable cost and service delivery system. However, using this approach, models can be updated as needed to reflect changes as the procedures are not difficult to conduct once the data has been collected. Consumers would certainly need to be forewarned of the possibility of such budget adjustments, however.

Fourth, the approach used here is called stepwise linear multiple regression. This means that it assumes cost changes in a linear fashion across the variables in the model. However, this may not necessarily be the case as the relation between these variables and cost may be more accurately described according to a different function (e.g., quadratic, cubic). While a linear relationship is a reasonable assumption to make in this case because it would seem that cost should rise proportionally as need for supports increases, there may be other relations that need to be explored to better predict cost. This notion can be addressed in future research.

Fifth, the consumers used in the present analysis were not randomly selected from the North Carolina CAP MR/DD population nor were we able to use data from the entire population served on this waiver. Rather, individuals were included because they had complete data records and were in the program for the entire year of the analysis. While a relatively large percentage of the consumers in the program were included in model development (47%), there nonetheless may be some bias in the data. Future uses of this approach must address this issue to produce the most accurate model. The model will be most accurate in predicting costs when the cases used to develop it accurately reflect the entire population of cases.

Sixth, while the final model developed in this study accounted for approximately 67% of the variance in consumer yearly CAP MR/DD program costs, an amount comparable with related research, this nonetheless means that approximately 33% of variability in costs is unaccounted for. Therefore, the model is not as accurate as it might be if the sources of this variability could be determined and added to the analysis. Future research must look more closely at the present variables to see how they might be refined to better reflect costs, and, must also look for other predictor variables that might contribute to the variability in costs across consumers. Based on this research, one variable that should be added, when available, is prior year's cost, as this variable seemed quite powerful for predicting costs in Evaluation 4.

Seventh, the standard to which the model was compared was actual yearly cost per person. While this is functional in the present circumstance, it assumes that current yearly cost actually covers the services that the person really needs and wants, that is, it is an ideal budget amount. To the extent that this is not true, using current costs may not be the best standard against which to compare the cost predictions of the model. Program administrators will have to determine if the current actual cost is the best standard for comparison, or, if some other standard needs to be applied. It would be prudent for future research to at least investigate if current costs adequately provide for individual wants and needs to best evaluate this standard of comparison.

Conclusions

Our first conclusion is that we believe that we were able to successfully replicate the approach to determining the amount of variability in individual consumer costs developed by Campbell and his colleagues. In fact, the approach should be easy to replicate for almost anyone as the procedures are very straightforward and the analysis relies on a commonly available and widely used statistical approach. While not replicating all aspects of their approach (i.e, particular measures used), we were nonetheless able to similarly select variables and enter them into a stepwise linear multiple regression analysis to produce a model that accounted for 67% of the variance in costs. This amount of variability accounted for is within the range found in the earlier work and suggests that this level of accountability may be what researchers might expect to find in systems where costs are not tied to particular personal or program variables in specific ways. Of course, in these latter types of systems of cost development, the amount of variability accounted for should be very close to 1.0 (i.e., 100%).

A second conclusion of this analysis is that this approach based on multiple regression does an adequate job of predicting overall yearly program costs. The residuals for most of the individuals in the program across all of our various evaluations tended to hover around 0 and, on the average, varied between $739 and $3,648 per consumer in each of the predictive evaluations that we performed. The size of these residuals would not appear to be insurmountable for using this approach to predict overall program costs. It is important to note that the model was most accurate (i.e., resulted in smaller residuals) when used to predict costs for individuals who, while not in the database used to develop the model, were nonetheless consumers in the CAP MR/DD program during the year used to develop the model. When using the model to predict scores in the following year, it was less accurate (i.e., resulted in larger residuals). Perhaps this reflects changes in the consumer variables over time or perhaps subtle changes in the service delivery system from year to year. Lastly regarding the predictive power of the model, when the predicted costs of the model for a subsequent year were compared with the individual's prior year program cost to predict their next year's cost there was not a significant difference between the resulting residual costs. If the predictive power of the model is no better than the prior year's cost, it suggests that it may not be worth the effort to develop and utilize this model when the costs of the prior year, which are readily available, may perform just as well in this regard. The limitation of this approach to budget development is, of course, that it would not work for people new to the system (e.g., people on a waiting list) as they would not have a prior year's cost data, and costs in a prior year may not match what is needed to meet the needs of an individual's person-centered plan.

Third, while the model developed in this analysis does a reasonable job of predicting overall program costs, as mentioned earlier it is notable that the model made some egregious errors in predicting costs for some individuals as there were residuals in each evaluation which were very large. Such residuals would have to be adjusted individually by the program and, of course, this adjustment process would require staff time and, hence, increased overall program costs. Additionally, this process of budget adjustment would likely delay consumer implementation of person centered plans because the size of their budget would be unknown. This problem of large residuals resulting from both under and over predictions of individual consumer costs must be considered by those evaluating the possible use of this approach because it is a serious issue that could add significant costs to a program in order to adjust the budgeted amounts for consumers whose predicted costs are in serious error. For example, across our evaluations we found between 8.9% to as much as 22.6% of the cases had residuals greater than $15,000, which certainly appears to reflect significant errors that would likely need correction. If these figures are extrapolated to the entire population of CAP MR/DD participants in North Carolina (6,194), it would mean that the system might have to somehow individually recalculate at least 551 and perhaps as many as 1,400 budgets in order to correct these large errors of the model. This number of adjustments would require significant costs in terms of program resources and take a significant amount of time to accomplish which might delay the implementation of consumer support plans. However, the number of adjustments needed resulting from the use of this model can be reduced by improving its accuracy. This can be done by adding additional variables into the model that capture some of the currently unexplained variance in actual costs. For example, Campbell and his colleagues have found in their research that the *ICAP*, the measure that they used to assess individual support needs, explains approximately 47% of their cost variance (Fortune et al., 2005) whereas in our model the measure of individualized support needs that we utilized (i.e., *NC-SNAP*) explained less than 1% of the variance in budgets. Therefore, identifying and including a more robust measure of individual support needs in our model would likely lead to a significant improvement in the accuracy of our model.

Unfortunately, we cannot compare the size of the residuals found in our evaluations to those that might result from the models developed by Campbell and his colleagues for we have noted only one instance where they have presented data regarding the size of individual residuals resulting from a systemwide application of their model (Campbell, 2002). In that report, residuals were potentially very large but did not reflect the application of the final model developed for use so we can't compare our outcomes with theirs. In their analyses they have tended to stress the amount of variability accounted for by their models (R^2), maximum predicted costs per variable in the model, and how the model can be applied to the data of a hypothetical consumer to demonstrate how to calculate predicted cost using the model. While they certainly note that not all individuals will fit a model well, they have not discussed exactly how to address these outliers nor have they discussed the possible increase in program costs that might result from the need to adjust budgets in cases where residuals are large. They have reported, however, that when their approach was implemented to create individual budgets statewide (Wyoming

– DOORS Model) there were no appeals to adjust predicted budgets (Fortune et al., 2005). We find this surprising, given the large residuals found in our studies. Perhaps merely knowing their exact budget and having the ability to make their own choices regarding expenditures proved sufficiently satisfying to consumers in that program.

In fairness regarding the size of residuals, we must note that the residuals that we found were likely larger than those that would result from the models developed by Campbell and his colleagues, for we did not exclude the data of as many individuals (outliers) as they did during the process of developing our model for predicting yearly costs. In the process of developing our model, we eliminated less than 1% of participants as outliers based on the inability of the model to result in a residual of less than 3 standard deviations from the mean of all of the residuals while Campbell and his colleagues (e.g., Campbell et al., 2005) have removed as much as 5% of their sample in developing their model. The result is that the predictive power of their final models are very likely greater than ours as their models have accounted for more overall variability than ours (67 vs. 88%), which should result in smaller residuals on the average. To test this possibility, we further developed our final model after eliminating enough outliers to achieve the 5% reduction in cases achieved by Campbell and colleagues. When we did this our model was able to account for 74% of the variability in costs. When we applied the model to the data used in Evaluation 2, average residuals were reduced from $739 to $383, suggesting that the accuracy of the model had indeed improved. Surprisingly, the number of cases with a residual greater than $15,000 was 52, one more than seen in our original analysis. So while the predictive power of the model was greater after removing 5 times as many outliers as in our original model, when it came to individual residuals, we found no difference. This is disconcerting as we would have to recalculate just as many budgets as with the previous model but would now have to create 5 times as many new budgets from scratch to provide for those eliminated as outliers.

In conclusion, we believe Campbell and his colleagues have created an interesting approach to predicting costs for people with developmental disabilities participating in publicly supported programs. It is easy to replicate, utilizing variables and a methodology that are readily available. It meets the goal of assigning costs to consumer in a consistent, objective fashion. Our research also indicates that the methodology is able to predict, with acceptable accuracy, overall program costs. However, we believe that the size of a significant portion of the residuals that resulted from our application of their approach suggests that it may be limited in terms of developing budgets for individuals. While those using this model in real world applications have reported that no individuals have appealed the size of their budgets, further explanation is needed nonetheless regarding residuals as the model insures that some people will be over-predicted and others under-predicted in terms of budget as the best fit regression line for all individuals is approached by the mathematics of the procedure. We therefore caution all who might be contemplating the use of this model for calculating individual budgets to utilize historical data that they have available to estimate the exact size of the residuals that might result from the application of the model in their circumstances in order to fully appreciate the number of potential budget adjustments that might be needed. If the size of the residuals is tolerable for the system, then this approach would be appropriate for calculating individual budgets. When doing this evaluation, it must be remembered that models developed in this process are only as precise as the variables that are available and entered into the model. Care should therefore be taken to enter variables into the analysis that prior research or experience has shown to likely be related to costs. Finally, from a research perspective, we believe that it would be useful for anyone evaluating this approach to developing individual budgets to present the actual residuals that result when using this model so that people might get a more accurate picture of how the model works in practice.

References

Bruininks, R. H., Hill, B., Weatherman, R. E., & Woodcock, R. (1986). *Inventory for client and agency planning.* Chicago, IL: Riverside Publishing Co.

Campbell, E.M. (2002). *2001 Individually-budgeted DD adult waiver model.* Pierre, SD: E = MC^2 Consulting.

Campbell, E.M., Fortune, J., Frisch, J.K., Heal, L., Heinlein, K.B., Lynch, R.M., et al., (2005). Predictors of expenditures in western states. In R. J. Stancliffe & K. C. Lain, *Costs and outcomes: Community services for people with intellectual disabilities.* Baltimore: Paul H. Brookes.

Campbell, E.M., Fortune, J., & Severance, D. (2000). Analysis of costs of services/supports for people with developmental disabilities in three states in the USA. *Journal of Intellectual Disability Research, 44,* 230.

Campbell, E.M., & Heal, L.W. (1995). Prediction of cost, rates, and staffing by provider and client characteristics. *American Journal of Mental Retardation, 100,* 17–35.

Cohen, J. (1988). *Statistical power analysis for the behavioral sciences* (2nd edition). Hillsdale, NJ: Lawrence Erlbaum Associates, Inc. Publishers.

Fortune, J., Smith, G., Campbell, E.M., Clabby, R.T., Heinlein, K.B., Lynch, R.M., et al., (2005). Individual budgets according to individual needs: The Wyoming DOORS system. In R. J. Stancliffe & K. C. Lain, *Costs and outcomes: Community services for people with intellectual disabilities.* Baltimore: Paul H. Brookes.

Building Wyoming Developmental Disability Waivers: Stewardship for the 21st Century

Clifford E. Mikesell, Administrator, Wyoming Department of Health, Developmental Disabilities Division

What Is Stewardship and How Can We Move Toward Better Stewardship of DD Service Dollars?

In 2002 Travis, Egger, Davies, and Mechbal called for concepts and critical issues that could move toward the better stewardship mentioned by the World Health Organization in their World Health Report 2000. They helpfully identified various important functions:

- Generation of intelligence
- Formulating strategic policy direction
- Ensuring tools for implementation: powers, incentives, and sanctions
- Building coalitions/building partnerships
- Ensuring a fit between policy objectives and organizational structure
- Ensuring accountability

The Wyoming Governor, Dave Freudenthal, in his 2003 budget address also called for better stewardship in the development and implementation of Wyoming state health service systems. These ideas are being pursued in Wyoming in the specialized health service area of developmental disabilities.

Saltman and Ferrioussier-Davis (2000) discuss the concept of stewardship in health policy as proposed in WHR 2000 and conclude that the concept "holds substantial promise if adequately developed and effectively implemented." The only other published article was an editorial in the *European Journal of Public Health* (McKee 2001) which also discusses the potentially major implications of the concept of "stewardship" of health systems, both for countries and for WHO as it seeks to strengthen its role as a credible advocate for global health.

Wyoming Department of Health Stresses Stewardship

Bob Peck, an experienced Cheyenne businessman, is familiar with the fears of business people over hiring people with disabilities (Peck & Kirkbride, 2001). Currently the Chief Financial Officer for the Wyoming Department of Health, he tackles stewardship in this way: What is stewardship? By Webster—the act of managing another's property, finances, or other affairs. For us—managing the monies entrusted to us by the state legislature and the federal government. How should we spend the funds entrusted to us?

- For the purposes intended
- Efficiently
- Cost effectively

What does the Wyoming Department of Health say about stewardship? It is important enough to include in our core values section of the 2005 Department Strategic Plan:

*"**Core Values:** We are **stewards** of the resources entrusted to the Wyoming Department of Health and value the responsibilities of that **stewardship**. We are committed to accessible, quality healthcare delivered in the most cost effective and efficient manner. We approach healthcare problems using scientifically driven evidence-based research. We communicate with the public, partners, and employees in an open and candid way."*

Toolbox for improving stewardship in Developmental Disabilities

Tools of stewardship include:

- Generation of intelligence
- Formulating strategic policy direction
- Ensuring tools for implementation: powers, incentives, and sanctions
- Building coalitions/building partnerships
- Ensuring a fit between policy objectives and organizational structure
- Ensuring accountability.

The Wyoming Department of Heath and the Office of Medicaid with the Developmental Disabilities Division are currently honing each of the tools.

Generation of Intelligence

Key questions in this domain of stewardship are "To what extent do developmental disability service system actors have useful intelligence at their disposal?" and "Do key actors have reliable, up-to-date information on current and future trends in waiver services and different aspects of waiver system performance, important contextual factors and actors, and possible policy options based on national and international experience with individuals with developmental disabilities?"

In pursuit of these goals the Wyoming Developmental Disability Division has pioneered Individual Budgets for waiver recipients (CMS, 2005). In 1999 Wyoming was the first state in the nation to begin publishing and posting survey reports of service providers on the Internet (http://wdh.state.wy.us/DDD/). In Wyoming, Decision Support System (DSS) software was implemented with the Office of Medicaid for fraud detection and pattern analysis. Program integrity was initiated with one team, and the Developmental Disabilities Division has recruited a second team for exploration of complaints and conducting investigations, site reviews, and financial inquiries that are followed up by either a CPA firm or the Medicaid Fraud Control Unit.

Formulating Strategic Policy Direction

This domain responds to the concern, "To what extent is there a clear sense of vision and strategic direction for the developmental disability system?":

- Is there clear articulation of developmental disability system objectives?
- Is there a clear definition of roles and responsibilities of public and private

actors in all four functions?

- Has there been a clear identification of policy instruments and institutional arrangements required to achieve improvements?
- Have the authorities developed strategies for making the required changes?
- Have they provided guidance for prioritizing developmental disability expenditures based on realistic resource and needs assessment and for monitoring effects of changes on performance?

As mentioned earlier, the entire Wyoming Department of Health has incorporated the values of stewardship in its 2005 Strategic Plan. Additionally, Developmental Disabilities outlines new possible directions such as the following exploration of support waivers for the Wyoming Select Committee on Developmental Disabilities.

New for 2000s

Centers for Medicare and Medicaid offer initiatives in the form of new waivers that allow more self-direction like:

- **President Bush's New Freedom Initiative**
  Money Follows the Person
  Real Choice Grants
- **Robert Wood Johnson Foundation**
  Self-determination Grants
  Cash and Counseling Grants

From this medley of new waivers Wyoming might consider adding a "supports waiver" that emphasizes giving individuals/families choice and control over a wide range of waiver services. Supports waivers operate under a fixed dollar cap on the costs of the waiver services that may be included in a person's service plan. About 14 states operate supports waivers (including Colorado and Montana). These waivers stress participant responsibility for managing services, including self-direction. The dollar cap under which these waivers operate ranges from $10,000 (Texas) up to $46,000 (Connecticut). The typical cap is about $20,000 with actual per capita expenditures generally running at 60-80% of the cap. These waivers are designed to support individuals who do not require or want the full range of services included in a state's comprehensive waiver. This additional waiver could have respite care and in-home support for birth through death for financially and clinically eligible applicants with developmental disabilities. The advantage of a family support waiver is that is could be written to have an average cost of $22,500.

Currently 78 children and 30 adults with developmental disabilities use these same services as part of the regular, traditional DD waivers. This new waiver choice could allow them and their families more satisfaction and freedom. It would allow the State of Wyoming to not ask for additional money and/or create a waiting list for the same number of people in the future.

Ensuring Tools for Implementation: Powers, Incentives and Sanctions

This domain addresses the concern "To what extent is there a regulatory framework that facilitates implementation of developmental disability policy, i.e., steers different actors in the desired directions?" "Regulatory framework" refers to the spectrum of rules, procedures, laws, codes of conduct, standards, etc., that exist. This will involve looking at the scope of existing regulation, conflicts or contradictions between stated policy and the regulatory framework (whether powers and responsibilities are matched) and the extent to which they are enforced.

In 2005 the Wyoming Legislature passed a state statute that allows the Department of Health to contract with waiver service providers and enforce civil penalties. Additionally, the Developmental Disability Division in conjunction with the Office of Medicaid wrote draft rules for the operation of the adult developmental disability waiver. Emergency referrals and case adjustment criterion have been determined and incorporated into our draft rules. Draft rules covering individual budgets, clinical eligibility, and exception care committee review procedures have been written with considerable input from key stakeholders.

Coalition Building/Building Partnerships

This domain addresses the concern "To what extent does capacity exist to create alliances of individuals, groups, or organizations for joint action around strategic health and health system priorities?"

Wyoming Developmental Disabilities Division has been active with the Governor's Council on Developmental Disabilities and the preschool and adult waiver service provider organizations. It has intermittently used an advisory council to gain additional input from stakeholders. One new tool that has been used for two years is extensive teleconferencing using interactive cable-based televideo conferences at up to 33 sites around Wyoming.

Ensuring Accountability

This is considered a separate domain at present on the grounds that it is a stewardship responsibility to ensure that all developmental disability system actors are held accountable for their actions. This will also contribute to consumer protection.

The Developmental Disabilities Division has contracted with Navigant Consulting, Inc. who conducted a cost study of the three home- and community-based Medicaid waivers in fiscal year 2004 and found a match of 97% of reported costs matched by waiver expenditures. Wyoming Developmental Disabilities Division is making every effort to use its dollars to serve the most people with medically necessary and essential developmental disability (DD) services across the state.

Increased documentation and active partnerships with the Office of Medicaid and the Wyoming Department of Health Fiscal Office has increased surveillance of exceptional care costs and requests for large rate increases. Fairness testing, adequacy testing, and expenditure sampling have been used to help ensure and enhance fair and appropriate reimbursement for waiver service providers. Electronic billing problems have been studied and provider satisfaction surveyed to increase provider appropriate payments. Extensive computer edits have been reinforced to allow for appropriate billing screening.

Ensuring a Fit Between Policy Objectives and Organizational Structure and Culture

This domain addresses the questions: "To what extent do organizational structures and management systems fit with policy objectives so that they help rather than hinder policy implementation?" and "To what extent have conditions been created by government that allow stewards themselves to be effective?"

Summary

In summary, there is much work to be done in the area of stewardship. There is further conceptual work to more rigorously characterize stewardship and delineate it from the overall concept of governance. There is analytic work required to explore the links between the organization and the operation of the stewardship function and different developmental disability system outcomes in different community settings. There is also a need to identify effective ways to strengthen the stewardship function in the statewide developmental disability system.

The work to increase stewardship has begun and requires continuous improvement efforts by the Developmental Disabilities Division. However, with constant vigilance it is possible to provide good care to the people we serve with our waivers and increase stewardship efforts at the same time.

References

McKee, M. (2001). The challenge of stewardship. *European Journal of Public Health, 11,* 122-123.

Peck, B. & Kirkbride, L. T. (2001). Why businesses don't employ people with disabilities. *Journal of Vocational Rehabilitation, 16,* 71-75.

Saltman, R. B. & Ferroussier-Davis, O. (2000). The concept of stewardship in health policy. *Bulletin of the World Health Organization, 78,* 732-739.

Travis, P., Egger, D., Davies, P., & Mechbal, A. (2002). Toward better stewardship: Concepts and critical issues. *Global Programme on Evidence for Health Policy Discussion Papers, 48,* Geneva: Switzerland: World Health Organization.

Specific Programs and Approaches

Working Together for Success: Enlisting and Training Staff in Dual Diagnosis

Ann R. Poindexter, M.D.

An absolutely essential factor in the development of successful programs for people with developmental disabilities and behavioral/psychiatric problems, no matter where they live, is the presence of excellent direct support staff. A number of factors are associated with maintaining this factor, including recruitment, training, and retention.

Recruitment of suitable staff members is felt by many to be a major problem. In addition to offering competitive pay scales, other factors can often be helpful. First, many agencies need to get away from the stereotype of youth being a necessity for employment—as well as male gender being an essential for working with individuals with significant behavior problems. (Many older women are quite successful in dealing with aggressive males with dual diagnosis.) Good employees are often a major recruitment asset if we ask them to tell others what they like about their jobs and to recommend others. Some agencies offer employees a bonus if they recruit/ recommend new staff members. Also, particularly in small towns and rural areas, getting the word out to groups that are interested in human rights/services, such as church and civic groups may result in good applicants. Background checks and random drug screens should be performed on all employees, without exception.

Hewitt, Larson, O'Nell, and Sauer (2005) acknowledge the importance of good job orientation but stress the importance of creating an intentional socialization process. They note that this process takes much longer than orientation, but should include welcoming activities, opportunity to understand the organizational history, values, and purpose, and immediate connection to a person in a similar role or to a mentor.

Secondly, staff training programs are another essential factor in maintenance of an excellent direct support staff. This training should, of course, provide all regulatory agency-mandated training such as first aid, CPR, personnel policy issues, privacy issues, etc. Also, general issues such as overall causes of mental retardation, general information about dual diagnosis, and general information about positive behavioral supports must be included. Specific medical issues concerning the individuals being served should be included, such as information about epilepsy, diabetes, cerebral palsy, and sleep disorders. General psychiatric information, particularly concerning depression and anxiety disorders should be included, even if none of the persons being served has a formal diagnosis of this sort, primarily because these conditions are exceptionally common and often missed in this population. Medication information, particularly concerning medication side-effects, should be included, with particular attention to the medications being received by the persons being served. Also, staff members should be specifically asked about topics they feel they need to learn more about in order to work successfully with the individuals being served.

Several interesting new protocols for performance- and competency-based strategies for training staff in methods of carrying out behavior plans and providing supportive and corrective feedback regarding observed performance in carrying out a behavior plan were recently outlined by Reid (2004). The steps for training staff to carry out plans include: describing each procedure to be carried out and providing a concise, written summary of each procedure; physically demonstrating how to carry out each procedure (typically in a role-play situation); having the trainee practice carrying out the procedure; observing each trainee's practice and providing supportive and corrective feedback; and repeating until the trainee demonstrates competence. After staff have been observed regarding performance in actually carrying out a behavior plan, Reid recommends that the feedback session be begun with a positive statement regarding the staff member's overall performance and specification of the procedures within the behavior plan that were carried correctly. Then information should be given regarding procedures within the behavior plan that were carried out incorrectly (if applicable), and specific precise instructions should be given about how to correctly perform these procedures. The staff person should be asked if anything needs clarification regarding the feedback presented or if there are any questions. The staff person should be informed about when his/her performance in carrying out the plan will be observed again. The feedback session should be ended with an overall positive or encouraging statement regarding the performance in carrying out the plan.

Crisis Prevention Institute (2002) notes five steps in debriefing staff after a crisis situation has occurred: 1) gather together as soon as it is possible and practical, but after everyone is back in control and all incident reports have been written; 2) establish the basic facts (What happened?); 3) talk about people's actions and feelings; 4) decide what to do next; and 5) give each other support and respect.

The training tools just described are designed to be used in a hands-on situation and are relatively time consuming, which some agencies feel is a problem. Retention of experienced direct support staff is a significant problem in all service programs for people with dual diagnosis. While the training curriculum they describe involved communication skills rather than specific technical information, Smoot and Gonzales (1995) found, while evaluating cost-benefits of a staff training program designed to improve patient management skills and relieve staff stress, that the trained unit had less staff turnover and staff members used less sick and annual leave than did the control unit.

Because of the scarcity of "live" training programs on clinical medical and psychiatric issues and the importance of day-to-day staff coverage issues, some type of self-directed instructional system may be of practical importance, particularly in community-based programs in rural areas. Piskurich in 1993 defined self-directed learning as a training design in which trainees master packages of predetermined material, at their own pace, without the aid of an instructor. He noted that the strengths of self-directed learning include availability when the training is needed, not when a class is being held; nonreliance on an instructor, which not only increases availability but decreases cost; on-site implementation, so trainees don't waste time and money traveling; and consistency of presentation, since self-directed learning packages present the same information each time they are used. Piskurich further notes that advantages for trainees include availability when the trainee is ready, trainee works at his/her own pace, individual choice of material, no surprises, immediate feedback, and provision of review and reference materials. Advantages for employers include multiple-site training, reduced meeting room cost, ability to capture knowledge of subject matter experts, fewer trainers required, reduced trainer travel costs, elimination of trainee travel costs, just-in-time training, downtime training, no training classes when busy, easier shift training, possibility of cross-training, training consistency, and less aggregate time spent. Self-directed instructional programs may involve paper-and-pencil, computer-based, and/or audio-visual formats. (NADD has available two CD-ROMs with a number of paper-and-pencil courses included, which can be obtained via the website www.thenadd.org. [Poindexter, 2003; 2006]). Various videotapes on a number of related topics are available from NADD as well as other sources. Objectives and quizzes could be readily developed for this type of material, thus broadening self-directed instructional offerings as needed.

As far as retention of staff is concerned, anything to decrease staff turnover rates should be considered. When problems arise, which they will, supervisors should not just cast blame, but should involve staff in developing a plan to prevent recurrence. The strengths of staff—the good things they do—should be reinforced consistently and often. Support staff should be involved in the development of all treatment programs, including the reasons for various treatment modalities. The major importance of staff in the success of treatment programs should always be emphasized.

Staff supervision should be positive, but not, of course, predictable. (Listening to staff is one of the most important tasks of a supervisor.)

References

Crisis Prevention Institute. (2002). *Staff debriefing strategies.* Brookfield, WI: Author (www. crisis prevention.com).

Hewitt, A. S., Larson, S. A., O'Nell, S. N., & Sauer, J. K. (2005). Orientation, socialization, networking, and professionalism. In S. A. Larson & A. S. Hewitt (eds.), *Staff recruitment, retention, & training strategies* (pp. 105-123). Baltimore: Paul H. Brookes Publ. Co.

Piskurich, G. M. (1993). *Self-directed learning: A practical guide to design, development, and implementation.* San Francisco, CA: Jossey-Bass.

Poindexter, A. R. (2003). *Self-directed instructional courses* (CD-ROM). Kingston, NY: NADD Press.

Poindexter, A. R. (2006). *Self-directed instructional courses: Young people with mental retardation/*

intellectual disabilities (CD-ROM). Kingston, NY: NADD Press.

Reid, D. H. (2004). Training and supervising direct support personnel to carry out behavioral procedures. In J. L. Matson, R. B. Laud, & M. L. Matson, *Behavior modification for persons with developmental disabilities: Empirically supported treatments.* Kingston, NY: NADD Press.

Smoot, S. L. & Gonzales, J. L. (1995). Cost-effective communication skills training for state hospital employees. *Psychiatric Services, 46,* 819-822.

Wyoming Works to Preserve Major Improvements in Retention by Enhancing Wages and Training

Robert M. Lynch, Kenneth W. Monfort School of Business, University of Northern Colorado; Jon Fortune, Clifford E. Mikesell, & Terry L. Walling, Wyoming Department of Health, Developmental Disabilities Division; and Kenneth B. Heinlein, University of Wyoming College of Health Sciences, Wyoming INstitute for Disabilities (WIND), UCEDD

Direct Support Professionals (DSP) in Wyoming provide guidance and support to more than 1,800 individuals with physical, psychiatric, and cognitive disabilities and other support needs. Wyoming, like other states, is challenged to keep DSPs in the field. In the 1990s this challenge was exacerbated by Wyoming's unenviable position of being ranked as 50th in the nation with regard to average and average starting wages of DSPs. (Braddock & Mitchell, 1992).

In 2002 the Wyoming legislature targeted a 28% increase in funding for Medicaid Home and Community-Based Services program for adults with developmental disabilities (and other programs supporting people with mental, physical, and health conditions). This increase in funding was specifically targeted to DSP compensation for the purpose of improving retention. The 28% increase in 2002 was followed with 3% increases in 2003 and 2004. With the appropriations, Wyoming's DSP wages were brought from 50th in the nation to above the national average. After the legislature made these changes Wyoming average wage rates for DSPs averaged $9.96 per hour as compared with $8.68 nationally, estimated from 37 state studies reviewed by Polister, Lakin, and Prouty (2003). Concurrent to the appropriation a study was commissioned to assess the impact of this intervention, conducted by the University of Wyoming, Wyoming INstitute for Disabilities (WIND), and directed by Ken Heinlein. The charts below show the wage changes for DSPs as a result of the action of the legislature in Wyoming and the associated effects of those wage changes.

Reimbursement and Retention of Wyoming Adult DD Direct Service Professionals

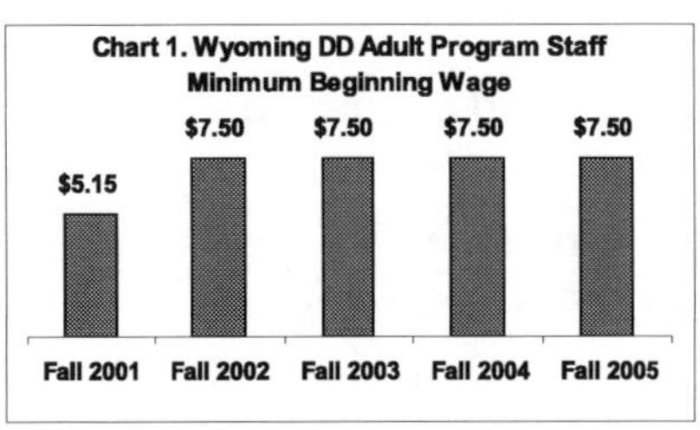

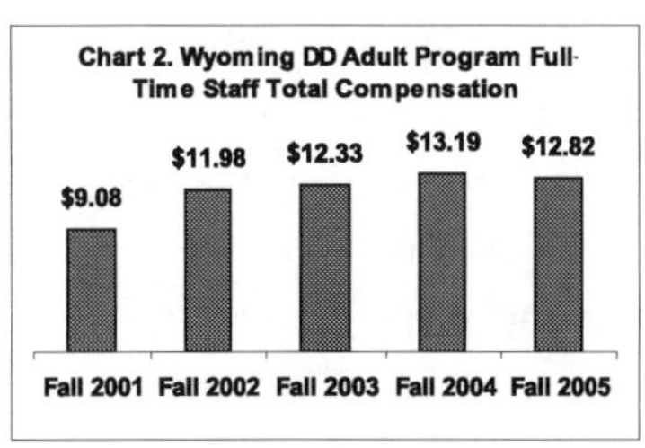

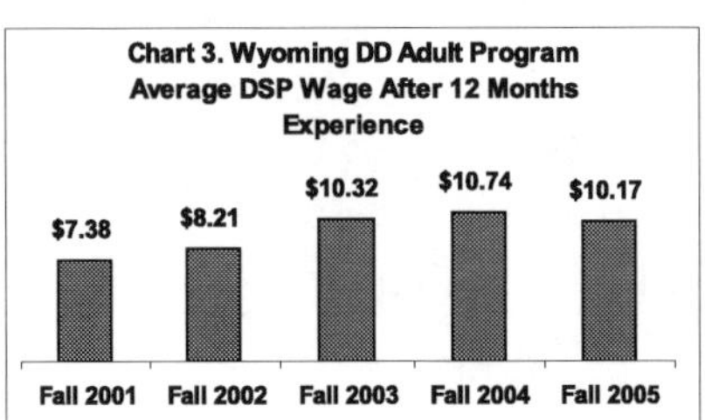

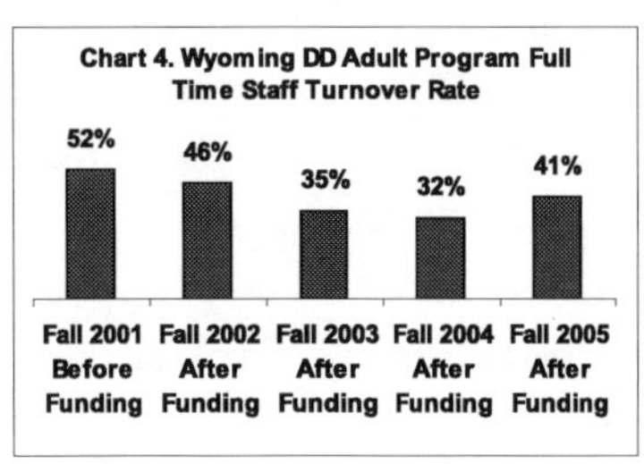

Following the decisive commitment of the Wyoming Legislature, as shown in Chart 1, beginning minimum wages of DSPs increased from $5.15 in 2001 to $7.50, slightly above the national average of $7.33 (Polister, Lakin, & Prouty, 2003). Between 2001 and 2005 the expenditures for full compensation (wages and benefits) for full-time DSPs increased from $9.03 to $12.82 (Chart 2); and wages for DSPs with at least 12 months experience increased from $7.31 to $10.17 (Chart 3). Associated with these notable overall improvements in compensation, the average annual turnover rate in Wyoming decreased from 52% in 2001 to 35% in 2003, to 32% in 2004. Turnover then climbed to 41% in 2005 when no additional cost of living increases were available (Chart 4). Economic boom conditions related to energy and mineral extraction also added to job competition in key regions across Wyoming. In the most recent year 10% more staff were hired and hours were worked to serve the several hundred people who completely vacated the state waiting list.

In 2002, the Wyoming legislature targeted a 28% increase in funding for Medicaid Home and Community-Based Services program for adults with developmental disabilities (and other programs supporting people with mental and physical health conditions). This increase in funding was specifically targeted to DSP compensation for the purpose of improving retention. The 28% increase in 2002 was followed with 3% wage increases in 2003 and 2004. With the appropriations, Wyoming's DSP wages were brought from 50th in the nation to above the national average.

Ongoing Training, Development and Recognition

The nearly 40% reduction in staff turnover cannot be absolutely tied to increased compensation. Wyoming also made a commitment to DSP training and career development. Wyoming is one of the first states to have a Direct Support Specialist National Apprenticeship program approved by the Department of Labor. The Ark Regional Services program in Laramie was one of the first apprenticeship sites in 2004. That program was based upon Ark's competency-based method of preparing DSPs through direct work experience and training with experienced professionals. Wyoming's Department of Workforce Services Director Kathy Emmons has called the apprenticeship program "an excellent way to build a targeted workforce to meet the needs of employers and consumers across the state of Wyoming." Wyoming's Gov. Dave Freudenthal has observed, "This program...effectively creates a career path for people to follow as direct support staff...This is a long-delayed recognition that this has always been a profession...It's fair to say that in the field of developmental disabilities, the direct support specialist has the most impact through direct contact with clients." Wyoming is also the first state to offer the Internet-based College of Direct Support (www.collegeofdirectsupport.com) for instruction of direct support staff. This initiative has resulted in over 100 graduates receiving certificates for program completion. More information is available at Wyoming's direct staff recruitment and retention web site: www.directsupport.org.

Wyoming has also made a major commitment to increase recognition of DSPs.

For three straight years Gov. Freudenthal has spoken at an annual awards banquet for DSPs in Wyoming. The annual award banquet honors eight recipients of the Direct Support Professional of the Year award, selected from nearly 100 nominees each year. The Professional of the Year awards are part of the "Do You Want Your Job to Make a Difference?" campaign, sponsored by the Wyoming Department of Health Developmental Disabilities Division, Wyoming providers of developmental disabilities services and the Governor's Planning Council on Developmental Disabilities. Reflecting on the Wyoming experience over the past four years, the Department of Health's Director Dr. Sherard observed that the legislation and training programs helped avert what was becoming a state crisis. "We were experiencing extremely high turnover in the position," he noted. "This is a position that requires training. By being able to offer higher wages and advanced training to those in the field, we feel we have a real cornerstone for success."

References

Braddock, D., & Mitchell, D. (1992). *National survey of staff compensation, turnover and related issues.* Washington, DC: AAMR

Polister, B., Lakin, K. C., & Prouty, R. (2003). Wages of direct support professionals serving persons with intellectual and developmental disabilities: A survey of state agencies and private residential provider trade associations. *Policy Research Brief 14*(2).

Specific Programs and Approaches

Telehealth in Rural America

John Holderegger, M.S., Kim K. Faulkner, R.Ph., Ph.D., & Theresa A. Faulkner, Ph.D., Mountain Regional Services, Inc., Evanston, Wyoming
Jon Fortune, Ed.D., Wyoming Developmental Disabilities Division, Cheyenne, Wyoming
Barbara Fortune, University of Wyoming, Wyoming Practice Residency

Introduction

In a general atmosphere of escalating healthcare costs and increasing consumer expectations, additional challenges arise when serving persons with complex needs in very remote settings. For example, in Wyoming, responding to these more general challenges is exacerbated by the long distances between service-delivery agencies involved and by the intemperate weather occurring throughout much of the year. Data from the 1990 United States Census Database provide a template for understanding the demographic, social, economic, and cultural landscape of Wyoming. The population of the state having the ninth largest land mass is numbered at 453,588, making it the least populated state, with the overwhelming majority of individuals living in rural and frontier areas. In an arena such as this, physically transporting specialized professionals to remote locations to render on-site treatment or quality training to workers in the field on subjects that are individualized and interactive is practically impossible. Coordinating and funding such efforts on any consistent basis is a logistically difficult, time-consuming, and expensive endeavor.

For these reasons, in Wyoming and elsewhere, there is an increasing interest in the use of telehealth as a means of healthcare delivery. Telehealth can be defined as the use of telecommunications technologies to provide health information and services. Moreover, recent technological advances have made this medium simpler to use and less expensive, both of which occur in a context of transmitting information with greater accuracy. Collectively, these factors further support the viability of telecommunications networking as an excellent means of providing services and doing so at a reasonable cost. Consequently, to meet these challenges in Wyoming, a pioneering telehealth project was begun in August 1995 in which specialists (in this case psychologists) make use of state of the art technology to provide statewide consultations from a single location to professionals and paraprofessionals dispersed throughout the state who, in turn, provide direct treatment services to individuals in sparsely populated settings.

More specifically, this ongoing project functioned to provide effective early interventions for individuals with developmental disabilities plus a psychiatric disorder. The initial aim of the project was to prevent decompensation among this complex group of individuals severe enough to require acute psychiatric hospitalization. By utilizing the State's compressed video network in conjunction with highly trained psychologists to orchestrate early interventions, it has become possible for individuals with dual diagnoses to avoid these more costly hospitalizations. This alone has saved millions of dollars and, more importantly, has assured a high quality, integrated life for persons with co-occurring disorders by allowing them to remain in their home communities.

However, since its initial inception, this telehealth project has gone two steps further, the second step having evolved into an additional service provided to the State's Division of Developmental Disabilities (DDD). First, it has been used to provide monthly statewide training modules for all participating compressed video sites on important topics such as active treatment and psychopathology. Second, it has been used as an expeditious route for timely referrals which allow more specialized assessment and treatment protocols to be implemented such that direct psychiatric hospitalizations can be avoided. Summarily, this technology furnishes a cost-effective way to 'bridge the gap' of distance while simultaneously avoiding delays due to inclement weather common in Wyoming during much of the year. In this chapter we will present data supporting how an integration of technology, the use of specialists in the field of dual diagnosis, and a telehealth format has been used to successfully address the more general and specific challenges in delivering health care services to individuals with severe needs.

Characteristics of Wyoming

Several factors make Wyoming the optimum environment for capitalizing on the benefits afforded by telehealth in general and more specifically for serving persons having mental health needs. In rural Wyoming, there is often a scarcity of resources for those seeking services from a mental health professional and large distances between psychological delivery sources (Butz & Recor, 1994). In most small towns, there are no mental health professionals to deliver services. Long driving distances and inclement weather combine with the mental health stigma in western society to make seeking such services prohibitive. Telehealth allows these services to be delivered to the persons in need in their own community by providing training to local staff who are in a tangible position to meet the needs of the person served. Few providers in rural areas (usually generalists), large distances between providers, insufficient knowledge of persons with developmental disabilities and co-occurring mental illness, treacherous winters, and expensive and difficult air travel precipitated the need to develop creative solutions for service provision in Wyoming.

When the telehealth project began, there were only nine providers serving 670 individuals; only two of those providers employed full-time psychologists to provide treatment to persons with a developmental disability and co-occurring mental illness. Today, there are over 400 providers of services to approximately 800 adults with a developmental disability. Still, only two of these providers have psychologists on staff, while a few others subcontract for psychological services from psychologists who are typically not specialized in treating persons with co-occurring disorders.

The Genesis of the Project

Under these contingencies, Wyoming's DDD was faced with the dilemma of devising a means of expanding the resources available at one of the community programs, Mountain Regional Services, Inc. (MRSI), where a cost effective and therapeutically efficacious program was already in place. Consequently, MRSI was asked by the adult program manager of the DDD to explore methods of providing consultation services to other programs where no psychological services were offered. MRSI's President and CEO, having had previous experience using Wyoming's Compressed Video Network, suggested the time slots available in the early morning hours, before college classes, could be used to provide consulting services via this networking system. Subsequently, MRSI psychologists began on-line consultation sessions via teleconferencing to the Regional Service Providers of Wyoming. The nature of the services required by participating agencies necessitated the implementation of two approaches to consultative efforts. These included a person-centered case consultation model and a consultee-centered educational consultation model, the latter for the purpose of providing education on selected topics relevant to serving individuals with developmental disabilities.

Services Provided Via Teleconferencing

In the person-centered case consultation model, a consultee encounters problems with a specific person they are serving. The task of the consulting psychologist is to identify and assess specific problematic behaviors, suggest a provisional diagnosis if this can be reasonably determined, then suggest intervention, treatment, and/or referral options. In the consultee-centered educational consultation model, the consultant focuses on the consultee and provides assistance with any difficulty the consultee has in performing his or her work role with the persons served. Examples include difficulties due to lack of knowledge, skills, objectivity, or confidence. In the latter case, it is common to find the staff member has the knowledge, skills, and objectivity required, but lacks confidence in his/her ability to carry out what is known.

Prior to the provision of person-centered consultations, providers are asked to supply the following information about the person served for use by the psychologist in preparation for the consultation meeting: age, level of intellectual functioning, DSM-IV diagnoses previously rendered, developmental history, history of institutionalizations, history/nature of physical and/or sexual abuse, normal daily routine, nature/quality of relationships with staff and peers (including differences if they exist), who is currently involved in the daily routine of the person receiving services, recent changes in the environment, current medication and any recent medication changes, types of behavior problems (antecedents and consequences of those behaviors), what has been attempted to manage the behaviors, and what was the outcome of each of the attempts, and any previous psychological evaluations available.

At the time of the actual two-hour consultation, all team members are asked to be present at the site. More specific data about the person receiving services can be elicited from the various team members. Then, a conceptualization of the problems and intervention recommendations of the person receiving services are provided. If necessary, follow-up consultations can occur to address incomplete symptom remission or less than acceptable improvement in behavior. Often, a second consultation is not necessary; rarely is more than a second consultation required to fine-tune recommended interventions.

Alternatively, in consultee-centered sessions, each compressed video site or multiple sites can simultaneously receive training in requested and/or relevant areas necessary for effectively treating persons with developmental disabilities. In addition, this model has another benefit in that issues of confidentiality encountered in the person-centered case consultation format do not have to be addressed, as no specific cases are discussed.

Assessment Outcomes

To assess consumer satisfaction, following each consultation or educational session, individuals attending were asked to complete a one-page evaluation form assessing helpfulness. Helpfulness was measured on a five-point scale ranging from 1 (definitely not helpful) to 5 (definitely helpful). Results indicated a mean rating of 4.6, falling between 4 (probably helpful) and 5. This finding was opined to support the notion that consultation services via teleconferencing were helpful. More specifically, consultees identified the following factors as contributing to their perception of helpfulness: 1) receiving factual information (e.g., what is psychosis?); 2) receiving specific recommendations (e.g., how do I reduce the aggressive behavior in this client?); 3) interacting with the consultant and their own teammates (e.g., group discussion and problem-solving); 4) interpersonal qualities of the consultant (e.g., interesting, keen observer, understanding, open to questions, good listener); 5) receiving an alternative viewpoint (e.g., a different way to look at or understand the reasons for the client's behavior); 6) getting feedback on their current practices or case conceptualization (e.g., we were giving consequences to an already self-punitive person, and we needed to be giving more praise); 7) the structuring of the consultation services (e.g., thorough, systematic, used examples, provided a focus, simplified the issues); and, 8) the specific benefits provided by the teleconferencing medium (e.g., visual contact, immediate transfer of information, cost effectiveness) (Faulkner & Faulkner, 1998).

Additional support for the positive outcome of the services provided came from administrative personnel directing Wyoming's Division of Developmental Disabilities (DDD). Data available to them indicated that none of the persons with a developmental disability served over the last four years by the DDD had returned to the state hospital. Moreover, only a very few had returned to the State Training School, with this being attributable more to overall medical than mental health concerns. In most other states, recidivism rates are typically much higher. This decline and its maintenance has been attributed to the added combination of teleconferencing services and the comprehensive evaluation services provided by MRSI.

How teleconferencing services have proven to be cost effective is further manifested by the progressively decreased number of consultations since the inception of the service in August 1995. The range of consumers helped, as well as a second demonstration of cost effectiveness, is attributable to MRSI's comprehensive evaluation services. This service is provided when consumers manifest intransigent behaviors or present as diagnostic enigmas that cannot be resolved because of the limitations inherent in teleconferencing. These consumers are referred to MRSI and receive a comprehensive evaluation on-site that ends when an in-person consultation is provided to representatives of the referring agency. In this way, more difficult cases receive specialized treatment allowing them to forego more costly psychiatric hospitalizations. Viewed collectively, outcome data collected from service providers and DDD officials support the notion that consultation and referral procedures utilizing a teleconferencing format has had a beneficial and cost-effective impact in the state of Wyoming.

Thus, telehealth has met our goal of providing effective early interventions to individuals with developmental disabilities and co-occurring psychiatric/behavioral distress before they decompensate to a level necessitating acute hospitalization. Utilization of the Wyoming State Compressed Video Network and services provided by highly trained psychologists has resulted in interventions capable of preventing hospitalization for all persons receiving services in Wyoming. Because of the effectiveness of this project, millions of dollars have been saved and persons with severe disabilities have been permitted to remain in their home communities. In fact, in the last five years of using statewide DDD telehealth conferencing, 90 individual consultations and 55 all-sites training sessions have occurred, with no consumer benefiting by the services later being admitted into the Wyoming State Hospital.

Impact of the *Olmstead* Decision

Such findings have a direct bearing on the compliance plans mandated by the Health Care Financing Administration (HCFA), (now CMS) in lieu of the landmark *Olmstead* decision and its far-reaching interpretation of the requirements of Title II of the Americans With Disabilities Act. As each state examines its institutionalized populations, the need for viable treatment options for individuals with mental retardation and co-occurring mental illness will become increasingly apparent. Defining the appropriate "least restrictive environment" for these individuals will present frustrating challenges unless service providers are capable of surveying existing programs and building comprehensive databases on current clinical and financial outcomes.

At the core of any systems analysis will be the issue of diagnostic capabilities available to a state upon which it can build a defensible system of referral, placement, and treatment. In this regard, Wyoming has created a unique center at MRSI, which provides in-house comprehensive evaluations as well as individual diagnostic consultative services via the state's community college compressed video network. Using a team of clinicians specialized in the diagnosis and treatment of persons with developmental disabilities and psychiatric/behavioral disorders, the Division of Developmental Disabilities uses both H.C.B.S. Waiver assessment funds and state monies to both identify potential consumers seeking services and improve habilitation services provided to current waiver recipients. As a result, the DDD had to create little in the way of new policies to develop its part of the *Olmstead* compliance plan and has yet to be involved with any legal action with regard to its placement decisions in this arena. Rather, Wyoming is directing its efforts at maintaining its most challenging consumers in community settings and expanding the capabilities of other provider agencies to increase their expertise in serving this most challenging population.

References

Butz, M. R. & Recor, R. D. (1994). *Rural psychology: Differences in culture, differences in therapy.* Paper presented at the annual meeting of the Montana Psychological Association, Great Falls, MT.

Faulkner, T. & Faulkner, K. (1998). Consultation via teleconferencing in rural Wyoming for providers of psychological services to the mentally retarded and mentally ill client. *15th Annual Conference Proceedings: Excellence from the Heart* (pp. 80-84). Kingston, NY: NADD Press.

Additional Recommended Information Sources:

Baer, L., Cukor, P., Jenike, M. A., Leahy, L., O'Laughlen, J., & Coyle, J. T. (1995). Pilot studies of telemedicine for patients with obsessive-compulsive disorder. *American Journal of Psychiatry, 152,* 1383-1385.

Baigent, M. F., Loyd, C., Kavanagh, S. J., Ben-Tovim, D. I., Yellowlees, P. M., & Kalucy, R. S. et al. (1997). Telepsychiatry: 'tele' yes, but what about the 'psychiatry'? *Journal of Telemedicine and Telecare, 3(Suppl. 1),* 3-5.

Ball, C. J., McLaren, P. M., Summerfield, A. B., Lipsedge, M. S., & Watson, J. P. (1995). A comparison of communication modes in adult psychiatry. *Journal of Telemedicine and Telecare, 1,* 22-26.

Blackmon, L. A., Kaak, H. O., & Ranseen, J. (1997). Consumer satisfaction with telemedicine child psychiatry consultation in rural Kentucky. *Psychiatric Services, 48,* 1464-1466.

Callahan E. J., Hitty, D. M., & Nesbitt, T. S. (1998). Patient satisfaction with telemedicine consultation in primary care: Comparison of ratings of medical and mental health applications. *Telemedicine Journal, 4,* 363-369.

Clark, P. H. J. (1997). A referrer and patient evaluation of telepsychiatry consultation-liaison service in South Australia. *Journal of Telemedicine and Telecare, 3(Suppl. 1),* 12-14.

Dongier, M., Tempier, R., Latinec-Michaud, M., & Meunier, D. (1986). Telepsychiatry: psychiatric consultation through two-way television. A controlled study. *Canadian Journal of Psychiatry, 31,* 32-34.

Duffy, J. R., Werven, G. W., & Aronson, A. F. (1997). Telemedicine and the diagnosis of speech and language disorders. *Mayo Clinical Proceedings, 72,* 1116-1122.

Graham, M. (1996). Telepsychiatry in Appalachia. *American Behavioral Scientist, 39,* 602-615.

Harrison, R., Clayton, W., & Wallace, P. (1997). Can telemedicine be used to improve communication between primary and secondary care? *British Medical Journal, 313,* 1377-1381.

Huston, J. L., & Burton, D. C. (1997). Patient satisfaction with multispecialty interactive teleconsultations. *Journal of Telemedicine and Telecare, 3,* 205-208.

Ioane, M. A., Bloomer, S. F., Corbett, R., Fedy, D. J., Gore, H. F., Mathews, C. et al. (1998). Patient satisfaction with realtime teledermatology in Northern Ireland. *Journal of Telemedicine and Telecare, 4,* 36-40.

Mahmud, K., & Lenz, J. (1995). The personal telemedicine system. A new tool for the delivery of health care. *Journal of Telemedicine and Telecare, 1,* 173-177.

McLaren P. M., Blunden, J., Lipsedge, M. L., & Summerfield, A. B. (1996). Telepsychiatry in an inner-city community psychiatric service. *Journal of Telemedicine and Telecare, 2,* 57-59.

Perednia, D. A., & Allen, A. (1995). Telemedicine technology and clinical applications. *Journal of the American Medical Association, 273,* 483-488.

Rural Psychotherapy and Developmental Disability

Judith Hill-Weld, M.S., M.F.T.

Therapy in the country is a lot like therapy in the city. People fall in love, they marry and divorce, fall ill, get healthy, gain and lose jobs, abuse alcohol and drugs, lose control of their anger, become depressed, worry, miscommunicate, parent poorly and well, find joy, and attempt to cope with the vagaries of life. Developmental disabilities and mental retardation in the country are a lot like they are in the city, too. Children get diagnosed, parents grieve and adapt, cope poorly and well. Teachers, doctors and behaviorists intervene and treat. The children learn and grow, develop more or less independence as adults, sometimes free of trauma and sometimes not. They find joy and frustration. And, in the country as in the city, some people do therapy and some people don't. However, as the fund of knowledge about providing psychotherapy to people with developmental disabilities grows, so too does the awareness of the unique difficulties and benefits of providing these services in a rural community.

I. What is rural?

This chapter describes the practice of psychotherapy within the context of a particular rural community. Nevada County is a 978 square mile area located in northern California on the western slope of the Sierra Nevada mountain range, stretching from the foothills eastward beyond the heights of Donner Summit and the cold blue waters of Donner Lake. As of January 2004, Nevada County was estimated to have a population of 96,100 (SEDD, 2004). Approximately 16,000 members of the population over age 5 have some kind of disability (www.FedStats.gov. , 2000).

The federal Office of Management and Budget and the Health Resources and Services Administration consider Nevada County to be a rural county. Adjacent Sierra County is distinctly rural, as are the sections of Yuba and Placer counties which share borders with Nevada County. Nevada County is considered part of Superior California, which is linked by the Northern Sierra Rural Health Network (NSRHN), a nonprofit corporation dedicated to the promotion of health and well-being of residents in rural northern California.

Alta California Regional Center (ACRC), a private nonprofit, contracts with the state Department of Developmental Services to provide support to over 13,000 people with developmental disabilities in a ten county area, including Nevada County. ACRC - headquartered in Sacramento - is one of 21 regional centers established by state law in 1969, and it maintains a satellite office in Grass Valley, in western Nevada County, and another office in Auburn serving the rural area of Placer County which abuts southern Nevada County. Alta California Regional Center serves approximately 400 people with developmental disabilities and their families in Nevada County, including infants at risk of developmental delay. The number of ACRC clients in Nevada County has increased over the past four years, as has the number of clients overall at the regional center.

Nevada County displays many characteristics typical of rural communities. Some of these include low level of population density, higher than state average percentage of owner occupied housing units, historical reliance on traditional rural industries such as timber and mining, and flight of young adults to areas offering greater employment or educational opportunities. To some degree, however, Nevada County may be atypical. For example, the percentage of the county's population that graduated high school and has at least some college is 15 points greater than the state average (SEDD, 2004). The percentage of the county's population subsisting below the poverty level is only 8.1% as compared to a state average of 14.2% (www.FedStats.gov., 2000), although the median income is quite similar to the statewide average. The unemployment rate in 2003 was 4.7%, much lower than the state average of 6.7% (SEDD, 2004). The number of people who report speaking a language other than English at home is only 6.4% as compared to a statewide average of 39.5% (www.FedStats.gov., 2000). The number of people residing in Nevada County who are 65 years of age or older is approximately 160% of the state average, while the number of children under age 5 is almost half the state average (www.FedStats.gov., 2000). The population of the county is growing, despite the fact that the numbers of deaths exceeds the number of births, indicating growth by migration (SEDD, 2004). The county's economy has, over the past decade or so, shifted to incorporate a heavy emphasis on tourism and the service industry, with the labor force dominated by management, professional, sales and office occupations (SEDD, 2004). Anecdotally, this writer has also observed two migration trends: One of families with young children moving to the area specifically in order to raise their families in smaller, slower-paced communities; the other of upper and middle-class retirees moving to the county to enjoy a rural lifestyle. A good portion of these families are supported by managerial/professional wages or retirement savings. Additionally, almost 28% of the population commute out of the county to work (SEDD, 2004).

The possible anomalies described above might allow us to describe Nevada County as somewhat "urban" in personality, although "rural" aesthetically, historically, and in official federal designation. The focus of this writing is the western part of the county, which contains the majority of the county's population (about 82%), particularly the population of persons with developmental disabilities.

II. What is psychotherapy and who is it for?

Psychotherapy is a mental health treatment that can take place in almost any location (e.g. home, private practice office, hospital, community care facility, community mental health center, doctor's office, mental hospital) and can be conducted by many different types of licensed clinicians (e.g., licensed Marriage and Family Therapist, licensed Clinical Social Worker, licensed Psychologist, psychiatrist). However, the psychotherapy model under examination in this chapter is individual, couple, or family treatment conducted primarily in the private practice office of an individual, masters level licensed practitioner. How does this model fit into the larger context of mental health treatment for people with developmental disabilities?

Clients appropriate for this kind of therapeutic setting generally suffer from cognitive impairment ranging from borderline intellectual functioning to the upper reaches of moderate mental retardation. Also, some individuals may have an autistic spectrum diagnosis, cerebral palsy, early childhood traumatic brain injury, or seizure disorder without broad intellectual disability but with significant challenges in adaptive functioning. The individuals participating in treatment generally must have the capacity to differentiate emotions, follow one-step causal relationships, have sufficiently stable memory from session to session, and be able to form a therapeutic alliance with the therapist. Clients with activated severe and disabling mental illness may not be appropriate for this type of treatment context; however, if an individual suffers with a chronic and severe mental illness which is successfully treated by other appropriate methodologies such as pharmacology, residual or contemporaneous issues may be effectively treated within this psychotherapy model. Individuals with excessive emotional or behavioral fragility may not be able to tolerate even the most carefully and gradually implemented psychotherapy. Also, individuals who are not capable of intentional behavioral choices, or who for some reason are unable to benefit from cathartic self expression, might not see lasting improvement from this type of psychotherapeutic setting. Individuals with lower level moderate to profound mental retardation are usually not served well by this model. Typically developing or mildly impaired parents, siblings, and other family members of persons with developmental disabilities are usually well-served in this model. The focus of such therapy is often to resolve emotional trauma, increase acceptance of the disability, improve anxiety management skills, or improve interpersonal communication. The psychotherapy may indirectly alleviate some of the symptoms of the disability but is not intended to treat the disability directly. Common diagnoses treated in this private practice context might include Adjustment Disorders, relational problems of many types, Post Traumatic Stress Disorder, anxiety disorders, depression, and bereavement. Many referrals, although not the majority, to this psychotherapy model result from problem behavior related to anger outbursts. Presuming appropriate medical evaluation and treatment has occurred, pharmacological interventions have been reviewed, behavioral analysis and methods of intervention have been implemented, some "anger management" issues are actually revealed to be connected to one or more of the common diagnoses listed above which has gone untreated. Therefore, "anger management" per se is not considered a diagnosis or judged as suitable for treatment until the pathway to anger is more clearly delineated.

Within the model described thus far, the specific method of psychotherapy depends to a great degree on the training of the psychotherapist. However, an ability to integrate both relational, psychodynamic approaches and cognitive behavioral treatments provides the clinician with the capacity to respond to a wider range of presenting problems and client disability levels. As described by other authors (Moses, 2002; Blotzer, 1999; Levitas & Gilson, 1999; Dosen, 2004), the orientation to therapy and the actual interventions must be carefully tailored to match the client's intellectual capacity, specific sensory strengths, learning style, and other individual needs.

Thus far this chapter has described a model of outpatient psychotherapy provided in a private, licensed, masters level practitioner's office which could occur in an urban, suburban or rural setting. The remainder of the chapter focuses on the specific challenges and benefits - for both clinician and client - of providing such a service in a rural community.

III. What makes the psychotherapy different in a rural community?

Imagine a first time gardener starting a vegetable garden at a new home at the distant end of a gravel road, ten miles outside of a town of 3000 people. What grows well here? Where can I buy fertilizer and seeds? Can I grow what my neighbor does? How much time do I need to spend in the garden if I grow everything I want to? How do I react when a plant fails to thrive? Who knows about soil amendments? Who can guide me in choosing organic alternatives to pesticides? When should I hire a professional? Would it be smarter to grow zucchini at home or just buy it at the market? Could I meet all my produce needs with my home garden? Should I use the square foot method? Raised beds? French double digging? Success at this endeavor is marked by the growing awareness of what you don't know and the minute accumulation of what you do. Accurate local information on the regional ecosystem and local mini-ecosystems is not served up in a neat and easy to locate package. To develop a comprehensive understanding of the entire network of resources requires a process of trial and error, observation, imagination, and careful cultivation of neighborly relationships.

Rural communities are often characterized by a system of decentralized, small-scale industries. The worlds of human service delivery and mental health treatment are no different. Despite the centrality of a county Department of Behavioral Health and a local branch of the appropriate regional center, the overall system for providing mental health services to people with developmental disabilities and their family members is fragmented, contains large gaps, and is sometimes inscrutable even to case managers and clinicians already working with the DD/MR population.

The public mental health system is strained to the maximum, with existing programs running at a financial loss. To conserve resources and apply them most effectively, this rural county is heavily focused on severe and disabling mental illness in adults, substance abuse treatment, and children with sufficient emotional disturbance to qualify for special education services. In addition, the county behavioral health system may sometimes disagree with the regional center about differential diagnosis of mental illness in persons with DD/MR. In fact, the county perspective seems to be that people with DD/MR don't often present as severely mentally ill, and more often are presenting "behavior management" issues (R. Erickson, personal communication, April 8, 2005). Those few people with DD/MR who are deemed to have severe mental illness and are otherwise eligible for county behavioral health services may not easily integrate with other county patients into typical treatment modalities, such as group therapy with non-disabled patients. Typical graduate curriculum for masters level clinicians does not include any component on DD/MR mental health issues, so the county has little opportunity to hire clinicians with this expertise. According to both regional center and county staff the current county caseload has "almost nobody" on it who is also a regional center consumer (R. Erickson, personal communication, April 8, 2005 and M. Mann, personal communication, March, 2005).

There is a statewide dearth of child psychiatrists, and there are none in Nevada County, in public or private practice. The county Behavioral Health department has two full time general psychiatrists and two part time contracted psychiatrists. There are no emergency inpatient facilities within the county for involuntary confinement, although county crisis staff will evaluate individuals in crisis as needed. The community is fortunate to have a few general psychiatrists in private practice. The regional center has contracted with a psychiatrist to provide medication management services two times a month in Grass Valley, but he provides no crisis intervention or psychotherapy services and periodically is unable to accept new patients.

Identifying the private practice mental health practitioners with interest and expertise in working with DD clients is complicated by the range of licenses in California and the opacity of insurance panel provider specializations. To develop a comprehensive understanding of the entire network of resources requires a process of trial and error, observation, imagination, and careful cultivation of neighborly relationships with a variety of professionals. Ironically, Nevada County has a large number (approximately 250) of masters and doctoral level licensed clinicians residing within its boundaries, although admittedly not all of them work locally.

ACRC contracts with "vendors" to provide assessment and short term counseling services when generic resources are not available. Given that direct federal reimbursement is not available for licensed Marriage and Family Therapists, and that contracts with county behavioral health entities are poorly paid, labor intensive, and decreasing in number, "generic resources" are generally not available. Additionally, because of the glut of psychotherapists in Nevada County, insurance panels are reluctant to accept new applications from clinicians, despite the panels' usual lack of developmental disability expertise. In Nevada County, three private practice psychotherapists and one agency are listed as vendors for counseling services to ACRC consumers. The reality is that two of the clinicians rarely if ever accept ACRC referrals, the counseling agency has a limited and relatively recent interest in this clientele, and the remaining clinician sees the vast majority of clients with developmental disabilities and mental health issues. That clinician, the writer of this chapter, maintains a caseload composed 50-75% of persons with developmental disabilities and their family members.

The regional center also contracts with behavioral consultants to provide functional analyses and develop behavior support plans. Few of these contractors have offices located within Nevada County. No licensed psychologists contracting directly with ACRC maintain offices in Nevada County, although at least one local licensed psychologist contracts directly with a residential care provider for consultation. ACRC staff and county Behavioral Health staff meet periodically and maintain a memorandum of understanding to help coordinate treatment. Their focus is strictly on persons with severe and disabling mental illness. There is no broad coordinated consultation network of local mental health professionals sharing expertise in DD/MR and co-occurring mental health issues.

In addition to the limitations of the greater mental health system, the rural community presents a tendency for the clientele themselves to be dispersed. If the population of Nevada County is approximately 96,100, with 30,050 located in the incorporated towns of Grass Valley, Nevada City, and Truckee, roughly 66,000 people reside in very low density areas (SEDD, 2004). Longtime rural families are often bound by "the ancient rule of neighborliness, by the love of precious things, by the wish to be at home" (Berry, 1990). Recent transplants move here to be closer to family, and/or because they crave the space, the trees, the privacy, the freedom to control their own few acres in the universe. People with even mild developmental disabilities may live permanently with their families in the country with inadequate public transportation to therapy, thus being highly dependent on parents, siblings, friends, or independent living skills instructors. In fact, due to funding cuts, regular bus service and dial-a-ride programs have recently consolidated investment around core corridors, cutting service to outlying areas by 18% in the past two years (M. Hill-Weld, personal communication, May 2005). They have fewer opportunities to access social experiences independently and cannot seek mental health help in privacy. Those who choose to move closer to town, in the more densely populated areas, have trouble finding affordable and appropriate housing.

Conversely, support services for people with developmental disabilities in a rural community are condensed and limited. Only three day-program facilities exist in western Nevada County (one is an adult day health care center) and at least one of these is often in precarious financial health. One of the day facilities (PRIDE Industries) also runs the largest independent living skills instruction service and a socialization program, so clients may be participating in this organization on multiple levels. Alta California Regional Center liaises with only six residential care facilities in this area. Two additional homes formally link to the nearby Auburn area in Placer County, although technically located in Nevada County.

Rural communities in Northern California are marked by two distinct mental health issues: consumer denial of need due to stigma and high rates of suicide (NSRHN, 2002). These mental health issues are then complicated by the infrastructure and resource issues described above, as well as rural geographic problems related to driving distances, poor roads and bad weather creating treacherous driving conditions.

Ethical Issues

Andrew Levitas and Stephen Gilson have said that "many people with MR live... in a persistent web of relationships in which their ability to change their perceptions and behavior is limited by the capacity of their caregivers (families, counselors, case managers, supervisors, or employers) to share or respond to such changes..." (Levitas & Gilson, 1999). In a rural community, the "persistent web" is densely woven, and there are only a small handful of webs for the entire community.

Rural communities present so many overlapping relationships and so few psychotherapy providers that the potential conflicts are great. For example, this writer accepted a referral for a group home client struggling with irritability and appropriate self assertion, but the client's primary need turned out be guidance and support in coping with the bullying behavior of his roommate. Six months later the roommate was referred to the same therapist, for entirely different issues. Despite the lack of overlap in presenting problems, the alliance with the first client was already formed - what if the bullying worsens and the first client wants to return to treatment? No other therapist was available locally at the time. There are also a limited number of large employers in the community, meaning - for example - the therapist could receive a referral for a client whose caregivers have a close professional relationship with a member of the therapist's family. If the therapist works with children, and has her own school-age children, the school districts are so small that the therapist could end up with child clients in the same classrooms as her own children, if she is not careful to avoid this overlap.

The "persistent web" also produces a higher than average potential for dual relationships. For example, parent advocates in any community who help run support activities for families coping with DD/MR also occasionally need therapeutic help. Being parent advocates they recognize the value of seeing a counselor with DD/MR expertise, but cannot work with the one therapist in town because they already collaborate with that person on the support activities.

Rural regions require greater than usual need for collaboration with care providers, especially for transportation: independent living support staff and residential service providers are particularly problematic because they are such a significant aspect of the client's daily functioning and can provide both important assessment information and can contribute to either the success or failure of treatment. While this dynamic occurs in urban areas as well, in a rural area there is even less opportunity to diversify the sources of support. The care providers also have no sources of DD/MR knowledgeable psychotherapeutic support for themselves, because there are not enough clinicians in the rural community to serve both the clients and the residential care provider or day program staff. These circumstances tempt the clinician to either excessively exclude care providers or to overly bond with them, almost treating them as clients. When there is an especially skillful and compassionate care provider, the psychotherapist may develop an idealizing transference and/or become more than usually invested in supporting that provider because she knows the value they contribute to the entire DD/MR community.

In a rural region with few DD/MR experts, the complex cases with a chronic history of behavioral analysis and management, pharmacological intervention, and medical evaluation often go to whichever professional is willing to spend the time with the person thinking about the problem. That means that referral to a masters level psychotherapist who works frequently and effectively with people with DD/MR may be tempting to case managers even if a licensed psychologist would offer more suitable expertise but practices outside of the local community.

Attempting to assess a person with DD/MR in their natural environs is exceptionally complicated in a rural community. Those who live at home may live in remote areas, thus challenging the mental health clinician's efficient use of time, or generating concerns about safety resources should the care provider or the client be less than warmly receptive. When there are only two or three day programs, and 50-75% of a clinician's private practice is DD/MR related, it is impossible to visit a client in their daily activities without potentially violating someone else's confidentiality or experiencing the challenge of juggling demands for attention from multiple former and current clients, including the client triggering the visit.

Counter Transference Issues

Of course, therapists bring an entire value system to the experience of doing therapy. Besides the existential anxiety described below, there are also political and social beliefs which impact the manner of treatment. For example, encouraging or even supporting person-first language or an increase in independent decision making when the individual's family or care providers do not share these beliefs, may result in the client's support system becoming angry and defensive. In fact, the client's presenting problem may be directly about the desire for greater independence from the family, thus posing the potential for a level of alienation from the support system which is intolerable for the client. While care providers can become angry and defensive in any size community, the difficulty is exaggerated in rural regions where the limited range and quantity of resources means the client may not have the option of developing an alternative support system.

This writer believes that a typical counter transference theme for therapists working with DD/MR issues is a desire to not feel any hopelessness associated with the permanence of a client's condition. Most of us, at some time or other, feel urgently compelled by our fear of hopelessness to view some component of a person's suffering as changeable and so to sometimes not accept the actual permanence of that condition, be it the retardation, the social skills impairment, the psychosis, or the personality structure created by early childhood abuse. However, in addition to this general and typical counter transference theme, psychotherapists in a rural community are also aware that the client cannot afford to continue problem behaviors that undermine employment, day program participation, or housing stability because they can easily run out of or use up local options. Combined with a lack of available clinicians, these issues may lead the therapist to pressure the client inappropriately for change, take on cases beyond her scope of expertise, or not acknowledge a poor client-therapist or poor client-care provider match.

Resolution of dependency with typically developing/developed clients can often incorporate the notion that therapy is a process and experience separate from this particular therapist. That is, the general population client ideally terminates therapy having integrated a new self and other object configuration generated by the positive relational experience of therapy, knowing that therapy and psychotherapists can be helpful and that he or she is capable of finding, getting, and using good help. The empowerment for future work lies within the client, not solely in this particular therapist. However the person with DD/MR, in addition to possibly not having sufficient autonomy skills - or adequate opportunities to develop these skills - also is stymied by the fact that there are either no or few other therapists with DD/MR expertise in the local community. The current counselor embodies both the literal assistance and the idea of help.

IV. What is the good news?

Private practice psychotherapy traditionally operates as an isolating and heavily boundaried experience. The combination of living and working in a rural area with the "persistent web" effect of the DD/MR community challenges that traditional model of individual private practice.

Just as that "persistent web" creates many challenges for the private practice clinician and the client, so it offers many beneficial opportunities, some immediately obvious and others more subtle and nuanced. Overall, though the familiarity with "the players" (i.e. the case managers, care providers, teachers, doctors, even friends) in a client's life can pose ethical and therapeutic challenges, it also supports a therapeutic shorthand. If the therapist can appropriately rely on successful past alliances with the members of an individual's support team to shift their approach to the client, or can utilize knowledge of the team's strengths and weaknesses in helping the client develop realistic expectations, the client may experience greater benefits from short term psychotherapy. Additionally, with clients who have mildly paranoid thinking or whose cognitive limitations may otherwise impact their perceptions of people, "familiarity with the players" might give the clinician a useful reality check. This reality check can work in both directions - for example, it can confirm a tendency toward paranoid distortions or anxiety dysregulation or it can validate the client's perceptions and focus the treatment on communicating wants and needs, strengthening coping skills, or even expanding the support team. For the client who needs a benign and supportive team to maintain the greatest possible level of independence, the clinician's skill at joining that team appropriately can help the client grow a greater sense of belonging, effectiveness, and self acceptance. Joining the team is easier when the therapist already knows the players and how to work with them effectively.

Some aspects of the "persistent web" can also benefit the clinician's skill development and professional satisfaction. For example, the constant potential for dual relationships and conflicts of interest challenges the therapist to develop finely honed ethical skills. Ethical decision-making becomes an active part of the therapeutic art rather than simply a form of polarized legal protection. In an age of increasing litigation, the ongoing effort to operate both therapeutically and to maintain the integrity of the profession grows a clinician's confidence and ability to assert her own boundaries more effectively and with appropriate degrees of flexibility.

The particular rural community discussed in this chapter offers some unique assets that benefit any therapist working with people with DD/MR. For example, although there is insufficient DD/MR mental health expertise, western Nevada County proffers an unusual breadth and depth of general therapeutic talent. This writer has discovered that regular consultation with a skilled colleague with a sophisticated background in psychoanalytic psychotherapy as well as many years of successful experience working within a short-term, managed care model provides excellent professional support. Using effective consultation can help bridge the lack of a professional network, at least temporarily until a network can be created.

Nevada County also has a kind of halo effect produced by the presence of the University of California at Davis's M.I.N.D. Institute 60 miles away. The MIND Institute is preparing to initiate a telemedicine project in Nevada County (and other rural communities), offering access to world class expertise in neurodevelopmental issues without the disruption of excessive travel.

Grass Valley is the home of FREED Independent Living Resource Center, a nonprofit working to support individuals primarily with physical disabilities who want to live independently. FREED has had profound impact on the perceptions of physical disability in this community, increasing the level of awareness and respect beyond what might be typical of such a sparsely populated area. Their emphasis on civil rights creates an atmosphere in which the right of people with DD/MR to seek out therapy if they choose could become more widely accepted. A local chapter of People First also contributes to the growing perception of people with DD/MR as human beings with emotions and opinions, not simply a collection of behaviors.

Nevada City houses the headquarters of the Northern Sierra Rural Health Network (NSRHN), which links together Superior California counties in efforts to strengthen access, coordination, and integration of health services for the uninsured and underinsured. The NSRHN collaborated with the Department of Developmental Services and the Far Northern Regional Center to develop a Telemedicine Access

Project (TAP) for consumers of DD/MR services. The TAP is designed to increase access to specialty healthcare and mental health services; although it was not designed to service ACRC consumers residing in Nevada County, it does provide a model for overcoming some of the barriers to mental health care present in rural communities. Additionally, the NSRHN, the California Institute for Mental Health and the California Mental Health Directors Association joined together in 2002 for a summit focused on "developing strategies to meet the mental health needs of California's rural north state." Their final report specifically mentioned the lack of clinicians willing and able to serve people affected by DD/MR. The reference to DD/MR reflects an increasing awareness of the mental health needs of this population. Finally, the NSRHN received grant funding to develop an integrated primary/behavioral health care model, in which the behavioral health clinician serves as a consultant and trainer to the primary care provider and offers short term intervention. While this model does not offer the full range of mental health services needed by people with DD/MR, it will help break down barriers of denial and stigma in a rural community particularly when a person with DD/MR may only be willing to see a primary care provider. If the behavioral health care clinicians obtain training in differential diagnosis for people with DD/MR, it may also increase the likelihood of early diagnosis of more severe mental health conditions.

The passage of two statewide propositions may offer positive impact on the awareness of counseling and therapy needs related to individuals and families impacted by DD/MR. Throughout California, the passage of Proposition 10, which emphasizes the health and well-being of children from age 0 to 5, may result in more children and parents receiving appropriate early intervention services for developmental delay. Broader early intervention could help identify families who need mental health counseling to develop acceptance of their child's delay or disability. The more recent passage of Proposition 63 (Mental Health Services Act [MHSA]) imposes a tax on the wealthy to increase funding for public mental health services in California by about 26% (Protection and Advocacy, Inc. [PAI], 2005). Because the new funds must support prevention and early intervention, education and training of mental health service providers, and innovative programs, the MHSA could help transform the entire public mental health system, including for people with DD/MR in rural communities.

The local regional center staff display extraordinary support for and insight about mental health issues and skillfully assess the appropriateness of psychotherapy for their consumers. They continue to coordinate efforts as much as possible with the county Behavioral Health Department and, with the recent passage of Proposition 63, may have the opportunity in a few years to participate in the development of innovative early intervention in mental illness.

Last, but not least, the parents of children and adults with developmental disabilities have galvanized tremendous support for each other, strengthening resource sharing, advocacy with the regional center and the school system, educating medical practitioners, and creatively generating additional social and recreational opportunities for their families. The willingness these families show to share disability information and provide support offers a natural means to disseminate greater awareness of the need for mental health treatment.

On a purely selfish level, with a nod toward the value of counter transference awareness, this writer acknowledges the great joy that comes from belonging to the "persistent web" and seeing a client's growth toward happiness, autonomy, and self realization. Although clinicians sometimes get this satisfaction in therapy, in a small rural community there are numerous opportunities to witness successes "by accident" which might not occur in an urban area. A therapist could take her own child to the local Little League field and coincidentally arrive in time to witness a game including two former clients, brothers, one with DD/MR, who six months ago were at each other's throats in constant conflict. Today they are gleefully passing the ball to each other and laughing at their mistakes.

Conversely, the therapist is also more likely to be exposed, by accident, to the "failures" and tragedies of her clients. In a rural community, the six degrees of separation are overt and remarkable every single day, in routine activities such as grocery shopping and eating at a restaurant. When a tragedy occurs, it is nearly impossible to avoid knowledge of it. Every car crash, crime, and fatality is described in the local newspaper. Simply standing in line at the grocery store can expose a clinician to conversations about clients' lives which she might not be privy to otherwise. Yet, this lack of protection-by-distance that private practitioners usually enjoy is strangely comforting. The psychotherapist is not functioning alone to rescue the client; instead they both exist within a world of people who know and see one another, where our struggles and challenges are not invisible, and where - despite the absence of a professional network - we do not have to grow the garden all by ourselves.

References

Berry, W. (1990). *What are people for?* San Francisco: North Point Press

Blotzer, M. A. (1999). The egocentric error. In R. J. Fletcher (Ed.), *Therapy approaches for persons with mental retardation.* Kingston, NY: NADD Press.

California Council of Community Mental Health Agencies (2005, March/April). From fail first to help first: Proposition 63 transforms California's mental health system. *The Therapist, 17* (2), 10-19.

Dosen, A. (2004). The developmental psychiatric approach to aggressive behavior among persons with intellectual disabilities. *Mental Health Aspects of Developmental Disabilities, 7,* 57-68

Levitas, A. & Gilson, S. (1999). Transference/counter transference in individual psychotherapy. In R.J. Fletcher (Ed.), *Therapy approaches for persons with mental retardation.* Kingston, NY: NADD Press.

Moses, K. (2002, October). Psychotherapy with older adults with developmental disabilities. *Conference Proceedings NADD 19th Annual Conference.* Kingston, NY: NADD Press.

Northern Sierra Rural Health Network. (2002). *North state rural primary care - Mental Health*

Summit: Collaborating for care. Nevada City: Author.

Protection and Advocacy, Inc. (2005). *PAI policy on use of Mental Health Services Act funds* Oakland, CA: Author.

Sierra Economic Development District [SEDD]. (2004). *Nevada County Economic and Social Indicator Review.* Auburn, CA: Author.

www.FedStats.gov. (2000).

Domestic Violence: Supporting Women to Live Safely in Community Settings in Alaska

Rebecca L. Bosek, Ph.D., Karen M. Ward, Ed.D., & Megan S. Wilts, M.S.

There is growing recognition that women with intellectual disabilities are vulnerable to exploitation and abuse. Compared to people without disabilities, they are at increased risk of psychological, physical, and sexual victimization (Curry, Hassouneh-Phillips, & Johnston-Silverberg, 2001). A history of sexual assault is a risk factor for repeated sexual assaults (Sobsey & Doe, 1991). Similarly, being a victim of other violent crimes is a risk factor for further victimization (Petersilia, 2000; Sobsey, 1994). Even when their victimization is identified and the need for ongoing services is recognized, women with intellectual disabilities often do not have equal access to systems designed to provide advocacy, intervention, and support. As a result, they remain at significant risk in home, employment, and community settings.

Women who have been victimized often lack an understanding of how to assess risk in relation to preferred activities (Sellars, 2002). They may have inaccurate information and misconceptions about sexuality and sex (McCarthy, 1999). As a result, they may develop boundaries that are blurred (Corbett, Cottis, & Morris, 1996). While some women avoid all contacts with potential partners, others engage in indiscriminate sexual behavior with multiple partners (Cruz, Price-Williams, & Andron, 1988). The women may have difficulties developing and maintaining positive sexual relationships (Stinson, Christian, & Dotson, 2002). Signs of sexual maladjustment include preoccupation with sex, excessive sexual conversations, and unusual sexual behavior (Matich-Maroney, 2003). Some women consider it appropriate to exchange sex for small personal items (Kaeser, 1992; McCarthy, 1999). Others view prostitution as an acceptable way to obtain emotional intimacy or as a form of legitimate employment (Bosek & Ward, 2003).

Witnessing domestic violence and a history of child abuse are risk factors for domestic violence, as women with intellectual disabilities become involved in dating and partnered relationships (Carlson, 1997). Some men view women with intellectual disabilities as compliant, loyal, and dependent; and these beliefs result in indifference toward their needs (Olney & Kuper, 1998). Women with intellectual disabilities may miss basic social cues or be unaware of how to keep themselves safe. They may remain in violent relationships because they do not want to be alone or have strong preferences to be in partnered relationships (Stromsness, 1993). It has been suggested that women with intellectual disabilities may endure oppression, exploitation, and abuse in exchange for maintaining a relationship with a male partner (McCarthy, 2002).

Perpetrators of domestic violence may be a date, partner, or spouse (Curry et al., 2001). Some women with intellectual disabilities are abused by acquaintances with disabilities after claims the two are in a committed relationship (Ward & Bosek, 2004). Also, women may be sexually exploited by peers without disabilities, due to beliefs that the perpetrators have authority over them (Mueser, Valenti-Hein, & Yarnold, 1987).

It is difficult for women with intellectual disabilities to leave violent relationships. When women have a history of victimization by family members, returning to live with the family may not be an option, thereby a source of potential support is not available (Carlson, 1997). Also, due to limited capacity and lack of resources, domestic violence shelters may not provide services to women with intellectual disabilities (Curry et al., 2001). The response of the criminal justice system to violent crimes against people with intellectual disabilities is generally considered inadequate (Petersilia, 2000; Sorenson, 2001). Available information suggests that the criminal justice system may not consistently intervene in domestic violence situations.

The response of the mental health system often results in additional trauma. The mental health symptoms of women who have been involved in domestic violence are similar to those of women who have been sexually assaulted (Carlson, 1997). However, women who have been involved in domestic violence frequently do not receive necessary counseling. Some professionals do not feel comfortable working with people with intellectual disabilities, while others apply generic interventions to all women regardless of the nature of their concerns. Professionals often lack the skills and training necessary to develop and implement specialized and adapted services (Mansell, Sobsey, & Calder, 1992). Finally, when women exhibit mental health symptoms as a result of both domestic violence and sexual assault, agencies often do not provide services addressing multiple issues (Zweig, Schlichter, & Burt, 2002).

There are multiple barriers that hinder the efforts of women with intellectual disabilities to extricate themselves from violent relationships. As a result, women who have experienced domestic violence are either not served or underserved. They remain at risk in home and community settings, as they form and maintain dating and partnered relationships. This article describes how specialized risk reduction and personal safety interventions can assist women who are dually diagnosed to live safely.

Key Components

In 1998, the Center for Psychosocial Development Clinic began to provide community-based support services for women who are dually diagnosed (intellectual disabilities and mental illness) and exhibit behavior that places themselves and others at risk. This agency is the non-profit service arm of the University of Alaska Anchorage Center for Human Development–A University Center for Excellence in Developmental Disabilities: Education, Research, and Service (UCEDD). Between 1998 and 2004, the women described in this article received services through the Clinic.

Description of the Population

Between 1998 and 2004, a total of 40 women were referred to the Center for Psychosocial Development Clinic. The majority of these women experience intellectual disabilities (90.0%) and mental illness (90.0%). Some of the women have Fetal Alcohol Spectrum Disorders (42.5%) and personality disorders (35.0%). Over a fourth of them have been diagnosed with Post-Traumatic Stress Disorder (27.5%). Over half of the women have been involved in relationships characterized by domestic violence (52.5%). The women range in age from 16-46 years old. Most of them reside in some form of supported living situation (90.0%), although a few women live independently in their own homes (10.0%). Less than a third of the women (30.0%) are employed in the community while the remainder are unemployed. All of the women are service recipients in agencies serving people with intellectual disabilities.

Risk Assessment

All women receiving services participate in a risk assessment. Information regarding domestic violence is obtained as part of the larger assessment process. Typically, at the time of referral, not much is known about either past or recent victimization or behavior that poses a significant risk to others. To obtain a comprehensive history, records are reviewed, discussions are held with the women, and collateral information is obtained through interviews with agency staff, guardians, and parents.

Also, several formal assessment instruments are administered. The Vineland Adaptive Behavior Scales (Sparrow, Balla, & Cicchetti, 1984) is used to gather information about overall adaptive behavior. The Reiss Screen for Maladaptive Behavior (Reiss, 1994) determines whether the women are displaying mental health symptoms. The Emotional Problems Scales (Prout & Strohmer, 1991) provides information about the women's current mental health and behavioral symptoms including anxiety, depression, withdrawal, sexual maladjustment, and self-esteem – symptoms often linked to a history of victimization. In some cases, the Trauma Symptom Inventory (Briere, 1995) indicates the presence of trauma-related symptoms. Finally, the Socio-Sexual Knowledge and Attitudes Test (Wish, McCombs, & Edmonson, 1980) assesses sexual knowledge along with attitudes regarding social and sexual practices.

Information provided by their risk assessments suggests that the majority of the women experienced a wide variety of mental health symptoms, including Post-Traumatic Stress Disorder. Also, they displayed risky social and sexual behavior that placed them at risk for exploitation and abuse. The women were impulsive and had a tendency to act without thinking through either possible risks or consequences for their actions. They frequented risky locations, carried on sexual conversations, and engaged in high-risk sex. Many of the women lacked knowledge about consent and were often touched without permission. Also, the women were known to touch others indiscriminately, make unwanted sexual advances, and assault others. Often, they lacked discretion when it came to forming dating relationships. Many women failed to make discriminations based on age or the nature of the relationship (e.g., stranger, friend, or romantic partner). They quickly formed committed relationships without determining whether the partner was safe. Often, the women chose partnered relationships with unsafe men such as sex offenders, and they experienced domestic violence and other forms of abuse. Finally, the women lacked knowledge about their legal rights and were unaware of community resources to assist them to remain safe.

Psychosocial Skill Training and Risk Reduction

Group psychosocial skill training is used to teach domestic violence prevention and risk reduction strategies. Information is presented to all women receiving services through the Clinic as part of a larger coordinated effort to assist women who pose a risk to themselves or others. The overall goal is to assist women with intellectual disabilities to live safely in community settings. Information about additional topics covered in the women's psychosocial skill training groups is available elsewhere and will not be repeated here (Bosek & Ward, 2003).

Group psychosocial skill training has several advantages conducive to working with women who are at risk. Being in a group assists the women to reduce isolation and loneliness as they begin to form connections with others. The consistency and predictability of group sessions provides ongoing opportunities for contact resulting in the development of female peer friendships, a much needed source of encouragement and support. When they hear their female peers disclose histories of victimization, feelings of shame, self-blame, and stigmatization are reduced as the women learn that others have gone through similar experiences. When they realize that female peers have managed to extricate themselves from violent relationships and do well, the women are provided with role models from their peer group. Feedback and modeling from peers who have gone through similar experiences is typically more readily accepted and valued than that provided by professionals or other authority figures. An unforeseen but valuable benefit is that the women know the potential dating pool and often share information on both safe and unsafe dating partners. On many occasions, women have been warned of the potential risks of dating certain men who have a history of violence and have chosen not to pursue relationships with them. Finally, group psychosocial skill training is a time and cost effective alternative to other therapies.

Psychosocial skill training includes several key themes for domestic violence prevention and risk reduction strategies including: 1) development of a common terminology and shared experience, 2) physical cues and feelings identification, 3) discriminations and timing, 4) public versus private talk, 5) safe and unsafe risks, 6) personal safety strategies, 7) social and assertiveness skills, and 8) legal rights and community resources. Psychosocial skill training groups are held weekly and last for 1.5 hours. Individualized Home-Based Services are provided for women whose intellectual functioning, mental health symptoms, or behavioral issues preclude their participation in groups.

Opportunities for Supervised Practice

People with intellectual disabilities typically retain information best if there are opportunities to learn, rehearse, review, and practice skills in the environments where they will be used. Once key themes for domestic violence and risk reduction have been presented during psychosocial skill training groups, the women are provided with opportunities to practice them in community settings. Depending upon the women's personal preferences and overall skill level, they participate in individual, paired, or group activities.

In all cases, the Center for Psychosocial Development Clinic staff assists the women to plan and implement activities. The staff provides support and feedback as the women choose an activity, coordinate information, make financial arrangements, and arrange transportation. During the activity, the staff asks questions about potential risks related to the activity, and the women are provided with opportunities to problem-solve specific strategies they could use to escape or avoid potentially risky situations. In order to increase generalization, questions are geared toward potential risks from strangers, acquaintances, friends, or dating partners. Throughout the activity, an emphasis is placed on personal safety regardless of the nature of the relationship, and an effort is made to teach the women to seek assistance from safe adults in the area, whom they may not necessarily know. Examples of these safe adults include a customer service representative, a store clerk, or a hostess in a restaurant. Once the activity has been completed, the staff is available to answer questions, to provide further feedback, and to discuss any concerns.

Outcomes

Outcome measures include pre-post tests of psychosocial skills to determine whether knowledge has been retained. Also, Center for Psychosocial Development Clinic staff maintain regular contact with staff from agencies providing other services to coordinate information and to collect other data, including incident and police reports. Also, the staff gathers written observations about the women's behavior in home, employment, and community settings to determine whether learned skills have generalized. Finally, focus groups are held with the women every six months to maintain the quality of risk reduction services, to determine overall satisfaction, and to follow recommendations for necessary changes, adaptations, and modifications to the program (Ward & Bosek, in press).

In the six years that we have incorporated domestic violence prevention and risk reduction services into our program, our outcomes include: 1) the two women involved in ongoing relationships with violent partners left these relationships with staff assistance, 2) none of the women receiving ongoing services established relationships with partners who had been identified as perpetrators of domestic violence, 3) none of the women had experienced additional rapes, 4) none of the women had legal charges of prostitution or other forms of sexual misconduct against them, 5) many of the women had experienced decreased supervision in home, employment, and community settings, and 6) the majority of the women had increased opportunities for social interactions with peers. Finally, both verbal and written feedback from focus groups suggests that the majority of the women are satisfied with services and current methods for teaching domestic violence prevention and risk reduction. These outcomes support the general efficacy of our approach to teach women to live safely in community settings.

Conclusions

Women with intellectual disabilities are vulnerable to situations involving domestic violence as they form dating and partnered relationships. Domestic violence prevention and risk reduction services provide a means by which women learn necessary skills to assist them to form safe relationships, as well as take the appropriate steps to keep themselves safe should they find themselves at risk.

References

Bosek, R. L., & Ward, K. M. (2003). Community-based support services for women who exhibit high-risk sexual behavior. *The NADD Bulletin, 6,* 3-7.

Briere, J. (1995). *Trauma symptom inventory.* Odessa, FL: Psychological Assessment Resources, Inc.

Carlson, B. E. (1997). Mental retardation and domestic violence: An ecological approach to intervention. *Social Work: Journal of the National Association of Social Workers, 42,* 79-89.

Corbett, A., Cottis, T., & Morris, S. (1996). *Witnessing, nurturing, protesting:*

Therapeutic responses to sexual abuse of people with learning disabilities. London, UK: David Fulton Publishers Ltd.

Cruz, V. K., Price-Williams, D., & Andron, L. (1988). Developmentally disabled women who were molested as children. *Social Casework: The Journal of Contemporary Social Work, 69,* 411-419.

Curry, M. A., Hassouneh-Phillips, D., & Johnston-Silverberg, A. (2001). Abuse of women with disabilities: An ecological model and review. *Violence Against Women, 7,* 60-79.

Kaeser, F. (1992). Can people with severe mental retardation consent to mutual sex? *Sexuality and Disability, 10,* 33-42.

Mansell, S., Sobsey, D., & Calder, P. (1992). Sexual abuse treatment for persons with developmental disabilities. *Professional Psychology: Research and Practice, 23,* 404-409.

Matich-Maroney, J. (2003). Mental health implications for sexually abused adults with mental retardation: Some clinical research findings. *Mental Health Aspects of Developmental Disabilities, 6,* 11-20.

McCarthy, M. (1999). *Sexuality and women with learning disabilities.* Philadelphia, PA: Jessica Kingsley Publishers.

McCarthy, M. (2002). Sexuality. In P. N. Walsh & T. Heller (Eds.), *Health of women with intellectual disabilities* (pp. 90-102). Malden, MA: Blackwell Publishing Co.

Mueser, K. T., Valenti-Hein, D., & Yarnold, P. R. (1987). Dating-skills groups for the developmentally disabled: Social skills and problem-solving versus relaxation training. *Behavior Modification, 11,* 200-228.

Olney, M. F., & Kuper, E. V. (1998). The situation of women with developmental disabilities: Implications for practitioners in supported employment. *Journal of Applied Rehabilitation Counseling, 29,* 3-8.

Petersilia, J. (2000). Invisible victims: Violence against persons with developmental disabilities. *Human Rights, 27,* 9-12.

Prout, H. T., & Strohmer, D. C. (1991). *EPS: Emotional problems scales.* Odessa, FL: Psychological Assessment Resources, Inc.

Reiss, S. (1994). *Reiss screen for maladaptive behavior: Test manual* (2nd Ed.).

Chicago, IL: IDS Publishing Corp.

Sellars, C. (2002). *Risk assessment in people with learning disabilities.* Bodmin, UK: BPS Blackwell.

Sobsey, D. (1994). *Violence and abuse in the lives of people with disabilities: The end of silent acceptance?.* Baltimore, MD: Paul H. Brookes.

Sobsey, D., & Doe, T. (1991). Patterns of sexual abuse and assault. *Sexuality and Disability, 9,* 243-259.

Sorenson, D. (2001, May). *The invisible victims.* Paper presented at the 2001 Arc

National Convention, New Orleans, LA.

Sparrow, S. S., Balla, D. A., & Cicchetti, D. V. (1984). *Vineland adaptive behavior*

scales. Circle Pines, MN: American Guidance Service.

Stinson, J., Christian, L., & Dotson, L. A. (2002). Overcoming barriers to the sexual expression of women with developmental disabilities. *Research & Practice for Persons with Severe Disabilities, 27,* 18-26.

Stromsness, M. M. (1993). Sexually abused women with mental retardation: Hidden victims, absent resources. In M. Willmuth & L. Holcomb (Eds.), *Women with disabilities: Found voices* (pp. 139-152). Binghamton, NY: Harrington Park Press.

Ward, K. M., & Bosek, R. L. (in press). Listening to women's voices: Risk reduction in community settings. *TASH Connections.*

Ward, K. M., & Bosek, R. L. (2004). [Demographics from a sample of women who are dually diagnosed and have been sexually victimized]. Unpublished raw data.

Wish, J. R., McCombs, K. F., & Edmonson, B. (1980). *The socio-sexual knowledge and attitudes test.* Wood Dale, IL: Stoelting Company.

Zweig, J. M., Schlichter, K. A., & Burt, M. R. (2002). Assisting women victims of

violence who experience multiple barriers to services. *Violence Against Women, 8,* 162-180.

Editors

John Holderegger, M.S.

Ann R. Poindexter, M.D.

Contributors

Jarrett Barnhill, M.D
Rebecca L. Bosek, Ph.D.
Kim K. Faulkner, R.Ph., PhD
Theresa A. Faulkner, Ph.D.
Barbara Fortune
Jon Fortune, Ed.D.
David J. Heath, M.P.A.
Kenneth B. Heinlein
Steven Hill, M.D.
Judith Hill-Weld, M.S., M.F.T.
John Holderegger, M.S.
Paul D. Kolstoe, Ph.D.
Edward A. Konarski, Jr.
Jim LeVelle, Ph.D.
Robert M. Lynch
Rebecca L. Mandal, Ph.D.
Clifford E. Mikesell
M. Chris Newman, M.H.A.
Jackie Olaveson, M.S.W., L.C.S.W.
Susan Orman, M.S.H.C.M., M.S.N., R.N.
Laurie L. Orvedal, M.S.
Ann R. Poindexter, M.D.
Rodney E. Realon
Marc J. Tasse, Ph.D.
Terry L. Wallking
Karen M. Ward, Ed.D.
Diane Wilson, L.C.S.W.
Megan S. Wilts, M.S.